THE FATS

THE FATS
WE NEED TO EAT

Essential fatty acids.
Feeling healthy,
Looking young

Jeannette Ewin

Thorsons
An Imprint of HarperCollins*Publishers*

Thorsons
An Imprint of HarperCollins*Publishers*
77–85 Fulham Palace Road
Hammersmith, London W6 8JB

1160 Battery Street
San Francisco, California 94111–1213

Published by Thorsons 1995
10 9 8 7 6 5 4 3 2 1

A catalogue record for this book
is available from the British Library

ISBN 0 7225 3166 4

Printed in Great Britain by
HarperCollinsManufacturing Glasgow

For my best friend and husband, Richard.

Acknowledgements

My thanks for help with this book go to Dr David Horrobin, whose research inspired its content, to Karen Wilson, for reviewing and commenting on the chapter concerning food supplements, and to Chef Mark Emmerson, of One Paston Place, Brighton, for reviewing the chapter on food and cooking. I also thank Professor D. Mark Hegsted, who gave me the most formative academic opportunity of my career.

Contents

chapter one

SETTING THE SCENE

As DNA (deoxyribonucleic acid – our genetic blueprint) dominated the medical news of the 1980s, so essential fatty acids will dominate the news of the 90s. Gatekeepers to the body's cells, essential fatty acids determine what can and cannot reach, or be transmitted from, DNA. The genetic material may contain the pattern, but essential fatty acids influence the final design. The degenerative diseases of the late twentieth century may not be because of 'mistakes' in DNA, but failures in the mechanisms which serve it.

This book is about the importance of fat – fat in our diet, and fat in our bodies. The very expression 'the importance of fat' may cause you to shake your head in disbelief, since fat is the antithesis of our modern idea of health and nutrition. However, there is another viewpoint. Without fat, no organ, no tissue, not one cell in the human body could exist. Fat in our food is essential for good health and long life.

The stars of this narrative are a particular type of fat – the essential fatty acids. The greatest applause goes to those fats described as omega-6, or n-6, fatty acids. Some important players in the cast you probably already know – linoleic acid, gamma-linolenic acid and their best known source, evening primrose oil. The omega-3 fatty acids, those much acclaimed components of fish oil, are also significant, but – as I shall explain – recent scientific evidence suggests that the omega-6 fatty acids have the more universal role in preventing illness and disability.

Fat is important

Fat in its various forms makes up approximately 25-30 per cent of our normal, adult bodyweight; and that most fragile of all organs – the brain – contains an even higher percentage. Fat cushions vital organs, provides a warming blanket under the skin, stores energy and serves as key building blocks in all living tissues. Adults need certain fats in their diet for tissue repair, and as basic constituents in chemical processes upon which depend energy, metabolism, reproduction and, ultimately, survival.

Some forms of fats in foods are more important than others. For example, children must have fat in their diets to grow and thrive. A clue about which fats are most important is provided by the interesting fact that mothers' milk is rich in certain essential fats – especially gamma-linolenic acid and its close biological relatives.

The link between fat and illness

Decades of warnings about our diet being responsible for the major killer diseases – most especially heart disease and cancer – have given fats a bad name. Medical concerns, social pressures based largely on current fashion trends, and effective marketing of low-fat products, have led many people to believe that the road to good health and a long life is fat-free. That viewpoint is not valid. The simple truth is that there are good fats and bad fats, and we need to know how to tell the difference. A good diet contains an adequate, balanced quantity of unsaturated and saturated fats. Even the much vilified substance, cholesterol, is a necessary element of life.

Western societies are plagued with a number of degenerative illnesses affecting an increasing percentage of the population, and a growing volume of medical evidence shows a link between this and diet. Research into the chronic degenerative diseases – cancer, rheumatoid arthritis, heart disease, rough and ageing skin, premenstrual syndrome and breast pain, osteoporosis, and various consequences of alcoholism – has pinpointed one common factor: and that is biological errors involving the essential omega-6 fatty acids.

Over the past decades we have heard much about miracle

molecules – DNA and proteins, and how they can be used to help identify and control the causes of disease. Now, medical science is telling a new story – a story about essential fatty acids, and how they actually regulate many key functions these other 'miracle molecules' perform. Essential fatty acids and their biological derivatives are the most exciting health and medical story of the decade. Learning to improve the quality of the fats we eat, and to use food supplements wisely, will make our lives healthier and longer.

A word to the ice cream and cake brigade

Don't be misled by this enthusiasm. Fats also cause trouble. Over time, too much fat in our diet, or too high a proportion of saturated fat in the foods we eat will cause molecular changes in our bodies that lead to premature ageing, debilitation and, eventually death.

Why read this book?

My primary objective of this book is to convince you that changing the types of fats you eat will help fade the spectre of illness. In my attempt to do this I cover a range of topics; including the basic biology of fats, the role of antioxidants in preventing degenerative disease, choosing a diet, using food supplements, and some cooking tips. As a somewhat separate issue, you will also find comments concerning medical research, how it is reported by the media, and the influence this reporting can have on our lives. Appendix c was written especially to comment on this subject.

Essential fatty acids and the future

By understanding how essential fatty acids function in the human body, scientists have laid the foundation for developing a new generation of medical products. These new drugs hold enormous promise. For example, repeated scientific investigations have shown products based on the omega-6 fatty acids can help prevent damage caused during radiotherapy, reduce the possibility of some serious complications of angioplasty (blood vessel surgery), help prevent osteoporosis, cure certain skin conditions, and prolong the lives of people suffering from pancreatic cancer. There is growing hope that these and similar compounds will eventually help alleviate the suffering of patients stricken with other forms of cancer as well. Even more exciting are early test tube experiments suggesting some of these new essential fatty acid derivatives may actually kill cancer cells without harming surrounding tissues.

Science has a human face

Over the years, the fatty acid story has not been a simple one. Good research always requires inventive ways to ask questions, and this frequently involves overcoming difficult technical problems in equipment and design. Some aspects of the fatty acids saga emerged only after the creation of wholly new types of equipment. For example, the development of a method of analysis known as gas-liquid chromatography allowed scientists to separate and quantify fatty acids in minute quantities of solution.

Other chapters of the developing fatty acid story depend on new insights into the metabolism of the human body. Many biological processes involving fatty acids occur in remarkably short periods. During the early stages of understanding these molecular interactions, scientists have to guess about what is happening. These guesses lead to new experiments, which lead to a better understanding, which lead to new experiments, and so on – until the puzzle is solved. It is not surprising that, in the often competitive fields of science, disagreements among members of the research community have led to some ideas being popularized and not others. Nonetheless, it is a painful truth that, no matter how popular an idea, if it is a wrong-turning it will lead those who follow it in the wrong direction. Until the right direction is found, no valid progress will be made.

Ultimately, science and discovery are about people, not machines, and much of the information in this book is based on the creative leadership and lifetime work of one man, Dr David F. Horrobin, co-founder and moving force behind Scotia Holdings Plc. Like so many great discoveries, the truth of his story springs from a gentle source. David Horrobin's most valuable tool in his search for a better understanding of health and disease is a simple and ancient flower – the evening primrose.

However, we begin this book, not with a story about a flower, but with a few words about David Horrobin's greatest mentor, and a most brilliant and irascible contributor to our understanding of human nutrition – Professor Hugh Sinclair.

chapter two

THE FATTY ACID STORY

IN the early years of the 1990s, two great thinkers were lost to the world of nutrition – Linus C. Pauling and Hugh M. Sinclair. Although one received wide international acclaim and the other did not, both contributed monumental insights into the workings of the human body and the foods it needs. These men shared a combination of characteristics setting them apart from most other scientists. Both were heretics, bravely holding beliefs vigorously denied by their contemporaries; and, both experimented on themselves, applying what they believed to be true to their own lives. Why are they linked here, in this book on fats? Because the work of one complements that of the other.

Hugh Sinclair saw the importance of molecules called essential fatty acids. These chains of carbon atoms, linked in places by structures called double-bonds, are highly susceptible to damage from a variety of sources, but most particularly from oxidation. They require antioxidant protection to retain their biological activity. Linus Pauling fought to explain the importance of vitamin C – a strong antioxidant in its own right, and a pivotal factor in maintaining the antioxidant activity of vitamin E. When essential fatty acids exist in a watery environment, they are protected by vitamin C; when their surroundings are fatty, or lipid, vitamin E takes over the role of protecting their delicate structures. One might say that those fine heretics, Sinclair and Pauling, shook intellectual hands over the structure of the carbon double bond.

To understand the fragile nature of essential fatty acids, it was first necessary to understand the fundamental nature of all molecules. Dr Linus Pauling, a double Nobel prize winner and campaigner against nuclear weapons, was the man who visualized and then described the structural organization of molecules. In his highly influential book, *The Nature of the Chemical Bond*, published in 1939, he described the parts of molecules and defined the basic rules about how they combine with one another. Through that understanding, he gave science a new view of matter, the elements it contains, and the nature of the interactions between molecules contained within it.

During his later years, Linus Pauling spent much of his time writing passionately about the importance of a simple, essential molecule in the human diet – vitamin C. Years before Pauling began his campaign informing people about its importance, vitamin C, or ascorbic acid, had been recognized as an essential nutrient, without which humans developed a disease called 'scurvy'. However, Linus Pauling advocated taking massive doses of the stuff; not a few milligrams, but several grams a day. He believed this powerful antioxidant made it possible for humans to withstand both disease and ageing.

Because Pauling's theories ran contrary to conventional medical teaching, he was vilified for what many saw as folly, and others regarded as dangerous. From most of his peers, Pauling's ideas met only ridicule. Eventually, as often happens in scientific heresy, during the last years of Linus Pauling's life his theories concerning vitamin C received credibility. Laboratory investigators discovered that a damaging form of molecule, known as a 'free radical', could cause significant harm to the genetic material and other substances in living cells. Antioxidants were shown to block the chemical activity of these rogue, free radical molecules, thus shielding more delicate molecules and subcellular structures against injury. The role of antioxidants in disease prevention became a popular theme for scientific study, and vitamin C was identified as an antioxidant with great medical importance.

In the light of what we are now learning about the significance of free radicals and antioxidants, it is arguable that Linus Pauling's fight for the recognition of vitamin C as a key factor in health may be as great as any battle he fought for the wider acceptance of the seemingly unacceptable. Linus Pauling's vitamin C was protecting Hugh Sinclair's fatty acids. Together, their theories could help us understand how to control certain killer diseases.

For Hugh M. Sinclair, the nutritional battleground concerned dietary fats, not vitamins. Sinclair believed small units of fat – essential fatty acids – held the answer to why western societies were enjoying higher standards of living, but suffering from increasing rates of certain degenerative illnesses. Like keystones in an arch, without these unique building blocks, the integrity of the whole is impossible.

It is easy to argue that the medical ramifications of Dr Hugh Sinclair's heresy are even more far-reaching than Linus Pauling's views regarding vitamin C. For his audience of established scientists, the complex nature and variety of conditions Sinclair attributed to specific fatty acid deficiencies seemed too fantastic to be true. Advancing decades saw people in developed countries achieve ever higher standards of living, and with better living standards came better diets and more food. Sinclair's theories met with amused curiosity. Was a deficiency in a foodstuff as ubiquitous as fat possible? And, if deficiencies did exist, how could they be responsible for medical conditions as diverse as osteoporosis, benign breast disease, and cancer?

Free radicals

Where do free radicals come from? Many are necessary parts of normal biological activity. Others, the real scourges of health in western society, are related to our modern lifestyle. Air pollution, cigarette smoke, the wrong kinds of foods, stress, exposure to X-rays, certain medications, too many vacation hours spent laying in the sun, excessive amounts of alcohol – all these create dangerously high levels of free radicals.

Following Hugh Sinclair's death in 1990, close associates wrote of his humanitarian work as a nutritionist in Holland in 1945, and shortly after that, his repetition of this work in the Rhineland. The governments of the Netherlands, the United Kingdom and the United States recognized and honoured him. In his memoir of Sinclair, his student and committed scientific follower, David F. Horrobin, wrote of Sinclair's two guiding principles that exemplified his research: first, to experiment on himself and, second, to think deeply, and to dare to follow through a line of ideas to its logical conclusion, no matter how amazing that conclusion might be.

Right and wrong conclusions about fat

Before going further with this story, I really should define my primary subject. Fat is a natural part of all living tissue and, therefore, being an organic substance, consists primarily of carbon, hydrogen and oxygen molecules. There are many different types of fats with differing characteristics; but, as a rule, all fats leave a greasy stain when pressed against blotting paper. Fats in foods provide a very rich source of energy: each gram containing about twice as many calories as the same amount of protein or carbohydrates. The many types of fats include cholesterol, wax, phospholipids and triglycerides. This last group, the triglycerides, are the most abundant in the body, and consist of one molecule of an oily substance called *glycerol*, and three fatty acid molecules. Obviously, much more will be said about fats and their biological significance in later chapters.

The scientific history of fats began more than a century and a half ago in Paris, France. In 1814, Michel Eugene Chevreul described the properties of fats and, two years later, isolated cholesterol from foods. At about the same time, other scientists in Europe identified the three primary elements in foods, which became known as carbohydrates, proteins and fats. For some time, fats were considered less important than the other types of nutrients because studies showed that dietary fat was not needed to produce body fat – for example, pigs fed an experimental diet containing only carbohydrates still gained body fat. However, as research continued, it became clear that not all animal species had the same dietary requirements. In some, a complete deficiency of fat led to disease and death. About that same time, the fat-soluble vitamins A and D were discovered, and diseases observed in animals on fat-free diets were recognized as deficiency symptoms caused by the absence of these substances.

But why were there no signs of essential fatty acid deficiency in the experimental animals used in tests leading up to the discovery of the fat soluble vitamins? It was because most of the early research on dietary fat was conducted using purified experimental diets containing rice or corn starch as their source of carbohydrate. It wasn't until later that nutritionists discovered both of these starches contain enough essential fatty acids, including the all important linoleic acid, to prevent deficiency diseases from this cause.

In the early 1920s, H. M. Evans, who discovered vitamin E, was joined in his laboratory by a young student, George Burr. Together they found that a purified diet of casein (the protein source), sucrose (carbohydrate), a mixture of salts, wheat germ, yeast and a small quantity of cod-liver oil caused young rats to fail to thrive and ovulate. More experiments also showed that about half of the experimental animals had kidney damage. This suggested the possibility of a new vitamin. Burr and his wife, a technician in Evans's laboratory, later conducted a series of experiments, using the same strain of rats and basically the same purified diet. Their findings led to the publication of two important papers, in which they described failure to grow, scaly skin, kidney damage, and impaired fertility. They concluded that a specific fat, linoleic acid, was an essential dietary ingredient. For some years to follow, essential fatty acids were erroneously referred to as vitamin F.

All of this was very exciting and satisfying, until soon after, when it was found that rats fed a diet containing quantities of arachidonic acid (a metabolic product of linoleic acid), in addition to adequate quantities of linoleic and linolenic acid, developed signs of essential fatty acid deficiency. Obviously, the subject of essential fatty acids was far more complex than expected. In fact, it was a subject full of technical minefields. For example, a few years later another scientist showed that, opposite to what George Burr and his wife had published, arachidonic acid is a much more powerful essential fatty acid than linoleic. Perhaps, it has been suggested, the original sample of arachidonic acids used by the Burrs had been destroyed by oxidation.

For those interested in the details of this story, I suggest you read from the master himself. In his introduction to what must be a classic book on fatty acid metabolism, *Omega-6 Essential Fatty Acids: Pathophysiology and Roles in Clinical Medicine,* by D. F. Horrobin, Hugh Sinclair tells the story of essential fatty acids as only someone involved in the story can. He tells us that in 1937, as a young man newly qualified in medicine, he visited H. M. Evans's laboratory and saw the work under way on the oestrous cycle. Sinclair had recognized that many western degenerative diseases were very rare in people living in poorer countries, and consequently proposed working on the role essential fatty acid deficiencies might have in causing a range of illnesses, including heart disease. His work was interrupted by World War II, but later continued at Oxford University, where, as the director of the newly formed Laboratory of Human Nutrition, he was joined by a number of outstanding young scientists to continue his work on essential fatty acids.

Early in 1952, Sinclair and his team of researchers were working on the problem of how and why cholesterol is deposited in the tissues of essential fatty acid deficient rats. Among this group, one man, Ancel Keys, held a different theory. Unlike the others, Keys believed all fats, including essential fatty acids, raised levels of blood cholesterol, and, in 1952 and 1953, he published two major papers stating his case. Here began one of the great debates in modern medicine.

Data from laboratories around the world were independently published contradicting Keys's conclusions. Nonetheless, Keys's ideas were those most widely accepted by the scientific community, and little time was given to work directed towards the cholesterol-lowering properties of essential fatty acids. One of his papers, using data on diet and blood-cholesterol levels from a number of countries, claimed to demonstrate a clear relationship between total levels of dietary fat and heart disease. In the excitement this paper created, very few noticed a response in the *Journal of the Statistical Society*. It showed that the material from which Ancel Keys had drawn his definitive information included data from 19 countries. Keys analysed data from only seven. By using all the data available, or by selecting another group of seven countries for his statistical analysis, different results would have been obtained, leading to other conclusions. As a whole, the data suggest that total dietary fat is not the most important influence in heart disease; some other factor is more influential. Sinclair believed that factor could be found in the specific types of fat eaten.

There are wonderful anecdotes about Hugh Sinclair, from both a personal and professional perspective. One significant twist in the fatty acid story involves a dead cat. Apparently

Sinclair was driven by such insatiable curiosity about the relationship between diet and health that he carried out postmortems on his family pets. In a memoir written after Sinclair's death, in 1990, David Horrobin tells how Sinclair and a student examined the tissues of a particularly old and exceptionally fat cat which had been pampered most of its life on cream and fish. To their surprise, despite its age, they found 'not a trace of atheroma'. (Atheroma is yellow fatty streaks and deposits on the inner lining of blood vessels, characteristic of atherosclerosis.) This, along with Sinclair's observations that Canadian Eskimos, despite living on a diet containing massive amounts of fat, have a very low risk of coronary heart disease, led to the conclusion that something more than linoleic acid, and its family of omega-6 fatty acids, was at play. The omega-3 group of essential fatty acids, starting with alpha-linolenic acid must also have a role. From a dead cat came a new line of investigation.

By the mid-1950s, Sinclair was convinced he was right about the causal role of both omega-6 and omega-3 essential fatty acid deficiency in degenerative illnesses. His scientific peers disagreed. Finally, in 1956, he wrote a long letter to the scientific journal, *The Lancet*, detailing his reasons for believing that unexplained 'diseases of civilization' are caused by deficiencies and metabolic errors in certain unsaturated fatty acids. The speculative nature of his letter received hot criticism, and led eventually to his being forced out of the Department of Biochemistry at Oxford University, where he was denied any further access to a laboratory. Nonetheless, he retained his Fellowship at Magdalene College and continued teaching there until his retirement. He was offered other positions, but decided instead to establish an independent Institute of Human Nutrition. Financial support for his work dried up.

For years, Hugh Sinclair remained in the academic wilderness. In 1985, just five years before his death, *Current Contents*, a review journal for scientific literature, described Sinclair's 1956 letter to *The Lancet* as a 'citation classic'. Sinclair's brilliant insight into the cause of degenerative disease had at last been recognized.

The evening primrose

A dynamic international pharmaceutical company, founded by one of his students, remains as a tribute to Dr Hugh Sinclair's achievements. In 1979, Dr David Horrobin, then Professor of Medicine at the University of Montreal, his wife Sherri M. Clarkson, Leslie Smith and Agricultural Holdings Company Limited (AHL) founded Scotia Holdings Plc. David Horrobin brought to the venture years of research experience into gamma-linolenic acid; while Sherri Clarkson and AHL added their knowledge of the evening primrose and the management of its seed production. Scotia Holdings Plc now operates worldwide with the aim of formulating, manufacturing, and marketing a range of products based on essential fatty acids and their medical properties. Today, the company produces many over-the-counter food supplements under the brand name *Efamol*.

New medicines based on the unique properties of essential fatty acids have been formulated and are progressing through the various stages of clinical trials. These target a variety of conditions including cancer, nerve degeneration caused by diabetes, and rheumatoid arthritis. Two of the promising products are a treatment for the side-effects of radiotherapy, and a drug that helps prevent blockage in arteries following angioplasty, or surgery on blood vessels.

The development of these products depends on oil from the seeds of a plant that probably originated in Central America 70,000 years ago – the evening primrose. The native Americans used the plant's healing powers by making a healing poultice from its leaves, and brewing a cough remedy from its roots. Botanists say the plant colonized all of North America, and from there spread to western Europe in ballast brought back on trading ships. Now, the plant has spread around the world.

The oil of the evening primrose is unique in its blend of essential fatty acids. Next time you are buying food supplements containing omega-6 essential fatty acids, think about this: Plant oils, including the ones we use in cooking, are obtained by extraction from the seeds, or – in the case of olives and avocados – from the nutrient substance around the seeds. Each seed carries its plant type into the next generation. To provide the singular blend of nutrients and energy required by the seed's tiny core – called the germ – to develop, the bulk of the seed comprises vitamins, minerals, proteins and carbohydrates. In addition, each seed contains fats as a concentrated form of stored energy, and to provide vital substances for early cell membrane development. To support plant growth until early leaves develop, every type of seed has a unique blend of fatty acids in its store of precious oil. Just as the singular form and characteristics of each variety of plant is determined by its genetic properties, so are the types and balance of fatty acids in its oil. When you buy a product containing borage oil, evening primrose oil or linseed oil, the number and balance of fatty acids it contains is determined by the type – or types – of seeds used in its manufacture. Evening primrose oil contains a small number of fatty acids.

Approximate fatty acid composition of selected oils

Fatty acid	Carbon structure	Olive oil	Evening primrose oil	Safflower oil	Borage (Starflower) oil
Palmitic	16:0	9.9	5.7	6.6	12.1
Stearic	18:0	2.6	1.2	2.5	3.5
Oleic	18:1	77.5	10.6	11.7	16.4
Linoleic	18:2	8.8	71.5	76.5	38.9
Linolenic	18:3		8.9	0.5	23.4

Note: Palmitic and stearic are saturated fatty acids; oleic is a mono-unsaturated fatty acid; and linoleic and linolenic are polyunsaturated fatty acids.

A word of warning. Recent investigations suggest that borage oil – which contains a proportionally higher quantity of gamma-linolenic acid than seed oil from the evening primrose – may not be a good choice as a food supplement. Although, per volume, it contains about twice the gamma-linolenic acid of evening primrose, research has shown it to be less effective. In addition, borage oil appears to have a negative effect on platelet aggregation, or blood clotting, which may be because of a toxic substance in the oil itself. All oils are made up of many individual types of fatty acids known as triglycerides. The chemical analysis of evening primrose oil shows it to be a simple blend, containing only four main fats. Borage oil, in contrast, contains a number of different triglycerides, including some that have received very little experimental investigation. It may be that one or more of these less known triglycerides give borage oil its worrying side-effect.

Natural substances can be as unhealthy as those manufactured in the laboratory, and research scientists are always vigilant about the safety of products available to the public. That is why methods are now being developed to extract only the gamma-linolenic acid from borage oil. This pure substance will have many future applications in over-the-counter and prescribed medicines.

How do essential fatty acids work?

Understanding what essential fatty acids do in the body, how long-term deficiencies can develop, and the medical conse-quences of these deficiencies, requires a brief biology lesson. Please read on.

chapter three

A BRIEF GUIDE TO THE
BIOLOGY OF FATS

Consider this: every moment of every day, billions of cells in your body are reproducing, interacting, repairing themselves, and conducting the biological functions prescribed by the specific chunk of genetic material responsible for their design. Inside each cell, a powerhouse of chemical activity is taking place. Molecules are being created, broken up, moved about and stored. Outside, in the separation that exists between cells, molecules of water and protein, minerals, vitamins, carbohydrate and fats pass by, interact, or stack up as part of an intercellular deposit. Nutrients and waste materials flow into and out of the cells' delicate membrane perimeters. Some molecules try to enter the cells and fail. Others bump up against membranes and stick. Messenger molecules bring commands from neighbouring cells or distant tissues – perhaps located more than a metre away. 'Make more of this.' 'Do less of that.' 'Contract.' 'Secrete.' Cells respond and change their intake and output of molecules accordingly. Everything is in a precisely tuned balance. Finally – sometimes within days, and sometimes after years of activity – each cell dies.

Figure 1 A simplified diagram of a cell

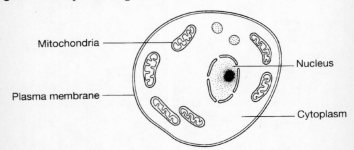

Life is a balanced flow of nutrients, waste materials and the products of biological activity, into and out of healthy cells. Building blocks for repair and the manufacture of molecules needed elsewhere in the body must flow into each cell in the quantities required. Biological messengers entering each cell must provide the information needed to know when and what to produce. Potentially toxic accumulations of each cell's waste products must be moved outside the cell and sent on their way to other parts of the body where they can be destroyed or discarded.

But, things do not always work smoothly. Infection, poor nutrition, and environmental factors, can alter the passage of these substances and change activities within cells. The result may be the premature death of cells, abnormal cell division and growth, or the production of the wrong substances for use elsewhere in the body. These are all circumstances that can lead to serious illness.

To understand how and why cells are damaged, it helps to think about their basic structure. As this book is about fats, our focus is on those parts of the cell containing the largest proportion of fatty acids. Cells have two main parts – an external wrapping, called a plasma membrane, and an internal, watery substance, called cytoplasm (*see Figure 1*). Within the cytoplasm, many small, sub-cellular structures, called organelles, busily carry out most of the cell's various activities – making new molecules, storing molecules, releasing energy for activity, and so on.

Why worry about sub-cellular structures? Because each plays a fundamental part in the biological activities of the human body. If the structure or function of any group of these particles is damaged, or fails to work properly, a healthy body can become a diseased body. That brings us to the subject of fat.

Each of the sub-cellular particles – the mitochondria for example – is constructed from a membrane, or biological 'mesh' of protein and fat molecules (*see Figure 2a*), and each has its own sphere of importance. The composition and structure of the membrane surrounding it control its function. Even the mighty nucleus, stuffed full of DNA molecules containing the genetic code, is wrapped in a lipid-rich membrane.

But, what is a membrane like? Plasma membranes surrounding

the cell consist of two layers of a fatty substance called phospholipid. Figures 2a and 2b give some idea of the complex nature of these layers. On the external part of the cell, the membrane has an electrical charge, and attracts water (hydrophilic). On its inner fatty surface, however, next to the cytoplasm, the membrane has no electrical charge – this surface is hydrophobic, and repels water. This difference is determined by the types of fatty acids in the membrane, and their attachment to molecules of choline (thought to be part of the B-vitamin complex) and phosphate. It is easy to see why this form of fat is known as a 'phospholipid', and why it is important to the transfer of molecules into and out of cells. For example, oxygen, fatty acids and steroids pass into the cell by first dissolving in the lipid components of its outer membrane. Transport of materials across cell membranes is also aided by the presence of large protein molecules, embedded here and there in the surface of this double molecular layer, which provide the water-filled channels through which certain substances enter the cell (*see Figure 2b*). These proteins also give the cell its immunological individuality.

The watery environment existing outside cells is filled with the coming and going of molecules, other cells and biological bits of 'this and that'. Between neighbouring cells, several kinds of tiny hormone-like molecules – called prostaglandins – stimulate activity. As an example, a white blood cell – with its flexible outer membrane edge pushing a path ahead of it while on its way to attack an invading bacterium – will slide over the cells lining blood vessels until it encounters chemical 'messengers' (known as eicosanoids, which include the prostaglandins) indicating the location of the invading organism. It then slides through the space between the cells forming the lining of a blood capillary, and out into the water medium beyond. Here, it may pass other cells, bump into passing molecules, even encounter other forms of scavenger white blood cells before it finds its prey which it will deactivate and destroy. By the way, the fatty acid molecules in the white cell's membrane help provide its fluidity, or flexibility, making movement within its environment possible. Polyunsaturated fatty acids can bend. That is one of their unique values.

Steroids and protein substances move about in the blood and

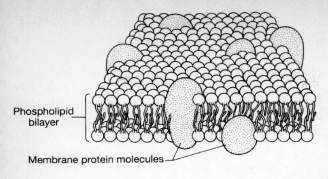

Phospholipid bilayer

Membrane protein molecules

Figure 2a A section of plasma membrane

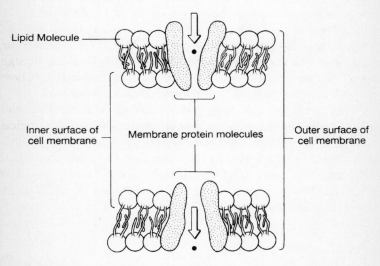

Lipid Molecule

Inner surface of cell membrane

Membrane protein molecules

Outer surface of cell membrane

Figure 2b Showing transport of molecule through cell membrane

tissues, controlling and changing the internal activities of the cells. If you are keeping a scorecard on fats, you will be interested to know that those steroids are a form of fat; as is their first cousin, cholesterol. And, the biological activity of those prostaglandins is largely dependent on the type of essential fatty acid they contain.

Not all cells enjoy close neighbours and a watery environment. Surrounding nests of cartilage cells, for example, a solid material containing elastic fibres fills the space. If the cartilage cells fail to maintain the chemical integrity of the substance around them, problems in joints can result.

And, in bone, the solid deposits giving it structure are constantly being dug away and restored by the cells it contains. We often think of bone as static, without much going on. In fact, bone is a hive of activity. Again, cells are located in clumps spread out in a solid environment. Channels connecting the space around cells run between the deposits of calcium and other minerals deposited in the solid substance of the bone. These deposits are always under attack by one type of cell, osteoblasts, and being repaired by another type, osteoclasts. Therefore, the local cells run the show; the mineral deposits are not permanent, and may become thick or thin under the influence of substances controlling the local cells. It is possible to imagine how degenerative changes in bone – osteoporosis, for example – can occur if the wrong messengers get to the cells in the bone, or if the bone cells are not functioning normally because of some internal flaw in their structure or metabolism.

Now, go back to the image you considered earlier of those billions of cells, working and acting together. Think how they are stacked up into tissues, and laced together into organs and limbs, including the heart, lungs, hands, nose, skin and nervous system, that combine to create the magnificently complex form you recognize in the mirror as YOU. Then, give a second thought to an old saying: *You are what you eat.*

It is all about nutrition

Every cell, every chemical interaction within every call, depends on nutrients supplied by the foods you eat. If your choices are good, everything works smoothly. If your choices are less than wise, and provided those billions of cells have a little too much of this – or far too much of that – trouble lies ahead. Sometimes your body can compensate for a short period. For example, there may be a supply of extra molecules of a key substance – a vitamin or trace mineral – stored away somewhere to cover requirements during a stretch of dietary imprudence. Or, the cells' chemical processes may begin to use a substitute for substances your diet has failed to provide. These and other responses to dietary deficiencies may carry you through short periods with no visible effect, if your food choices improve.

If, however, you simply fail to give your body what it needs, look out for problems. There are essential nutrients the human body cannot make for itself. If these essential components of food are scarce, or totally denied for a period, the body ceases to function normally.

The fundamental connection between diet and disease has been known for 200 years. Back when men still went to sea on a diet of dry biscuits and bad meat, their officers saw a link between the foods the men ate and outbreaks of debilitating illness. Limes and lemons prevented scurvy. Cereal grains kept pellagra at bay. Although it took many decades to identify the exact substances involved – vitamin C and the B-vitamin, niacin, respectively – medical science was on its way to understanding the importance of nutritional deficiencies.

Nutrition has come a long way since the days of limes and scurvy. We now know that the human body consists of five major classes of chemicals – proteins and amino acids, carbohydrates and sugars, fats and lipids, water, salts – and a complex blend of genetic material. All these substances are necessary in the functions of life, which include movement, growth, reproduction, digestion, metabolism, and respiration.

Every schoolchild is told that he or she needs a daily diet containing a good balance of proteins, carbohydrates, vitamins and minerals, all mixed with a good helping of water. They know that protein builds muscles, is necessary for the repair of cells, and is important for a variety of chemical activities including the production of hormones, antibodies and enzymes. And, it is almost certain that students understand carbohydrates are important for energy. But what about fats? Most of us believe fats are bad for us: real killers. In fact, fats are absolutely vital for normal growth and good health.

What fats do in the body

People often think of fat as those substances that leave oily smudges on paper serviettes, or spots that are hard to wash off clothes. Most of us give fat little regard as an important part of our basic nutritional requirements. But, fat is a vital component of living organisms, and although some forms of fat are manufactured in the body from excess calories we consume, there are other fats we can only obtain from the foods we eat. If our diet does not contain the right balance of these substances, we run a significant risk of developing degenerative illnesses. Why is this so?

Fat facts

Body fat, the kind we gain after eating too many calories, has several basic functions – it stores energy, helps protect the kidneys and other organs, and serves as a warm blanket of insulation under the skin. More important, however, are the more subtle roles for fat. Fat molecules aid the absorption of vitamins A, D, and E from the gut. They are vital parts of the bile salts produced by the liver to aid digestion of fatty foods. The core structure of steroid hormones and cholesterol, which perhaps surprisingly is a necessary substance in a healthy body, consists of fat molecules. And, fats form part of every membrane in every cell in the body. An insufficiency of the fats we need can lead to illness.

There are two sources of fat – plants and animals. Animal fats are mainly saturated, although oily fish, like herring and halibut contain higher proportions of unsaturated molecules. Animal fats are found in all forms of animal protein, including cheese, milk and eggs. Vegetable fats are usually oils, and these contain a high proportion of unsaturated fatty acids.

There are several different types of fat found in the body. These range in size and complexity from the simple fatty acid (the real subject of this book), through the more complicated lipoproteins, like those found in cell membranes, to the rounder, larger molecules of cholesterol and steroid hormones.

A word about cholesterol

Rightly or wrongly, cholesterol has become a major 'bogy-man' in medical lore. The truth is that cholesterol is absolutely necessary for good health because it:

- is the core molecule in steroid hormones, including sex hormones;
- forms part of lipoproteins in cell membranes;
- is needed for the formation of bile salts;
- helps transport fats around the body; and
- forms part of fat soluble vitamins.

There are two sources of cholesterol in the body. A small amount comes from foods such as eggs and cheese, but most is made in the liver, especially from saturated fats.

Few medical stories are as complex and confusing as that regarding blood cholesterol and heart disease. There was a time when doctors saw red flags when an individual's total blood cholesterol rose above a certain level. Shortly thereafter, two forms of cholesterol were recognized: LDL-cholesterol (Low Density Lipids) – which contains large amounts of saturated fats – and HDL-cholesterol (High Density Lipids) – which is rich in proteins. Statisticians found LDL-cholesterol to be closely linked with the risk of heart disease; and now research suggests that the HDL variety appears to actually help strip off deposits from the walls of blood vessels.

If you sit down and read the literature, you will find there is another important player in this saga of fats and heart disease – blood triglycerides. And beyond that, essential fatty acids control both the cholesterol and blood triglycerides. There are chapters still to be written in the heart disease/lipid saga, but the smart money is on essential fatty acids emerging as the heroes of the piece. Arguably, the most important fats in the body are the essential fatty acids.

What are fatty acids?

What stands out in any good diet book is a list of essential nutrients; this should contain vitamins, minerals, names of specific amino acids and other substances such as fibre and water. If the book is very good, it will also tell you to eat foods containing certain types of unsaturated fats. The human body cannot produce for itself all these 'essential' substances, molecules and compounds – they must all be obtained from our diet.

Essential fatty acids – the specific unsaturated fats our bodies cannot manufacture – are the wands of the gatekeepers that allow other molecules to pass into and out of the billions of cells that make up all the tissues in our bodies. This flow of molecules takes substrate, or working material, to a cell's genetic material for replication of chromosomes. It provides food and building blocks for cells to use in their own repair and in the manufacture of proteins and other substances that need to be carried elsewhere by the bloodstream. And, this flow of molecules, screened by the same essential fatty-acid rich configurations within cell membranes, allows the passage of waste material from the cell to be carried away for disposal.

There is some disagreement about the definition of the term 'essential'. For the purist, the same rule applies to fatty acids that is employed for other nutrients: 'essential' is limited to the description of necessary nutrients that the body cannot manufacture for itself. When this rubric is applied to fatty acids, only linoleic acid can be classified as an omega-6 'essential'. (Among the omega-3 fatty acids, alpha-linolenic is the one most frequently regarded as 'essential', because the body can produce others from it.) Justification for this position is drawn from the fact that linoleic acid is found in large quantities in the foods we eat, and that it is the starting point for a series of metabolic reactions that produce a series of other, more biologically active, molecules we know as the omega-6 fatty acids. From linoleic acid, the metabolic processes of the human body produce gamma-linolenic acid (GLA), this is further changed to form dihomo-gamma-linolenic acid (DGLA), which is later used to form arachidonic acid (AA), from which adrenic acid and certain prostaglandins are formed.

However, there is another viewpoint. Any disruption to the normal processes of metabolism, which involves linoleic acid and its derivatives, is potentially dangerous. Figure 3 shows the pathway of changes from linoleic acid to some of its important metabolites. Notice that two biological catalysts, or enzymes, are involved: delta-6-desaturase and delta-5-desaturase. A number of external factors can destroy the activity of both enzymes, and thus make it difficult – or even impossible – for the body to convert linoleic acid to gamma-linolenic acids and its biologically active metabolites. If the action of these enzymes is blocked in the body, then it is necessary that these fatty acids be supplied by other sources. That means linoleic acid and all its metabolites are *essential fatty acids*. Because it is believed that the same series of enzymes affect the metabolism of both the omega-3 and omega-6 series of essential fatty acids, factors blocking the production of biologically active molecules from linoleic acid are also thought to be responsible for blocking the metabolic path from alpha-linolenic acid.

Scientific research, over the past several decades, has identified a surprising number of problems that can arise during the body's conversion of linoleic acid to gamma-linolenic acid, and during the further metabolic processes for which gamma-linolenic acid is a precursor. Writing in the journal *Progress in Lipid Research*, in 1993, essential fatty acid expert Dr David Horrobin said that 'A substance should be described as an *n*-6

Figure 3 Omega-6 and omega-3 essential fatty acid metabolism

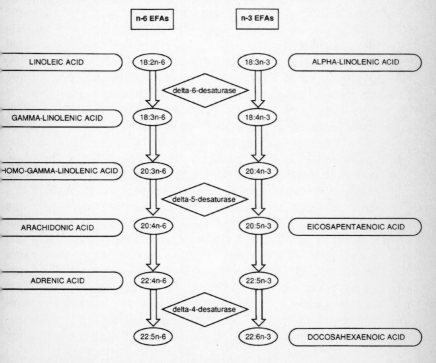

EFA [omega-6 essential fatty acid] if it is both present in food and if it can reverse the biological and biochemical features which result from the exclusion of all *n*-6 EFA from the diet.' To underline the validity of this statement, research has shown that linoleic acid, gamma-linolenic acid and arachidonic acid can all reverse the symptoms of essential fatty acid deficiency. All are found widely distributed in foods in small amounts. Arachidonic acid is found in meats, egg yolk, fish, fish oils and other sea food. Gamma-linolenic acid is found in oats, barley and in small amounts in a variety of common foods. Since these fatty acids are found in food, and can reverse all the features of linoleic acid deficiency, they should be regarded as essential fatty acids.

Both gamma-linolenic acid and arachidonic acid are found in important amounts in human milk. This is not only an indication of their importance to human growth, but also their significance as essential fatty acids. Recent tests have shown a significantly lower quantity of essential fatty acids in the structure of the grey matter brain tissue from babies fed formula when compared to tissue from breast-fed infants. Because the brain is one of the most rapidly developing organs during early life, it is likely that essential fatty acid levels in early life help determine long-term health in an individual.

A fatty acid is a simple molecule containing the same carbon, oxygen and hydrogen included in other nutrients, only in a different arrangement. They are called 'acids' because each molecule includes a particular carbon-based structure of atoms (-COOH) that can change into an ion, or radical, under certain conditions. The word 'acid' should not be a worry, however, because the acidic properties of these molecules are small.

The best way to visualize a fatty acid molecule is to think of a string of pearls, where each pearl is a carbon atom. At one end of the string is a clasp: this is the end that hooks on to other molecules, including glycerol in triglycerides. When a fatty acid exists alone, without a connection to another atom, it is called a free fatty acid – its 'clasp' end is made up of a sub-molecular 'clump' containing a carbon atom, two oxygen atoms and a hydrogen atom – which together are called a carboxyl group, as was mentioned earlier. At the other end, the string of pearls stops with a clump of atoms consisting of a carbon atom and three hydrogen atoms, together known as a methyl group. This is the business end of a fatty acid molecule and – in combination with the total number of pearls, or carbon atoms, in the string – what happens from the methyl group back to the 'clasp' determines the fatty acid's activity.

In foods, the length of the chain of carbon atoms in the fatty acids which are dominant in a product influences many of its characteristics, including taste, the way it responds to hot and cold temperatures, and its smell. Foods, such as butter, which contain a predominance of butyric acids and other short-chain fatty acids, are firm to the touch when cold, but soften quickly when exposed to room temperatures. Cocoa butter, extracted from the seeds of the cacao plant and used in chocolate, is also rich in short-chain fatty acids, and melts at body temperature. Beef fat, which is high in stearic acid, and which contains a chain of 18 carbon atoms, becomes very firm in cold temperatures, and remains hard at room temperature. Next time you wash up after enjoying a beef steak for dinner, notice the characteristics of the fat left on the plates. Sometimes the unique qualities of a fat have commercial use; for example, early candles were often made from beef tallow because it burns well, but remains solid at room temperature. Today, the flavour and appearance of many commercial food products, such as crackers, are improved by coating them with blends of certain oils. While this processing trick adds to the product's attractive features, it also creates a source of hidden fat, which few people recognize.

Because different length fatty acids have different characteristics, both the flavour and the sensation of eating foods vary according to the fatty acids that dominate them. Pie crust made with lard tastes and smells different from that made with butter or vegetable oil. In part, beef gravy does not taste the same as chicken gravy because of the presence of stearic acid in one, and not in the other.

Before leaving the subject of fatty acids in foods, it is important to mention that an animal's diet has a direct influence on the fatty acids it deposits in its tissues. There is substantial evidence to show that many artificial feeds produced for large animals grown for market change the ratio and types of fatty acids stored in their tissues. Other differences take place as well, but the fats are most remarkable. Usually, these changes influence the taste and smell of products that end up on our dinner table. Perhaps easiest to recognize is the difference in the taste and smell of chicken raised on a diet of corn from that of birds of identical breed raised on artificial feed.

Saturated versus unsaturated fats

The second characteristic which separates groups of fatty acids is their degree of saturation. Let us think again about that string of pearls mentioned above. Then, think about the fact that – in scientific jargon – carbon atoms have a valance of four – that means that each carbon atom can 'hook on to' four other atoms. These 'hooks' are called bonds, and it is natural for all four bonds to be completed between the carbon atom and another carbon atom, some other single atom, or part of a second molecule. Nature demands that all of these 'hooks' hold on to something else – rather like hands clasped. If a break should occur, and one of the 'hooks' becomes incomplete, that position will be filled almost instantaneously by a passing atom or molecule.

In a saturated fatty acid all of the 'hooks' are complete, and there is no room for any other atom or molecule to attach itself to the carbon chain. That means that all of the pearls, or carbon atoms, are using each of their four 'hooks' by attaching to the two neighbouring carbon atoms on either side, and to two hydrogen atoms. These are rigid molecules, with little bend. In fat, such as dripping and butter, they are firm, or hard, when placed in the refrigerator.

But what happens if some hydrogen atoms are missing? The fatty acid molecule is then 'unsaturated', and adjacent carbons form double bonds between each other. Instead of sharing one hook, they share two. A fatty acid may have one double bond (point of unsaturation) – as in oleic acid – or several. Linoleic acid has two double bonds (*see Figure 4*), and gamma-linolenic acid has three. These points of unsaturation are extremely important to the biological activity of a fatty acid. All essential fatty acids have two or more points of unsaturation. These are the working parts of the fatty acid because they form the basis

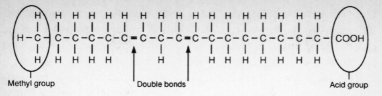

Figure 4 Showing the two double bonds in the linoleic acid chain

for 'lock and key' relationships with other biologically active molecules. Equally important, these double bonds bend, and give shape to the molecule. These 'bendy bits' also provide flexibility. It is this characteristic of unsaturated fatty acids that, when incorporated into a cell membrane, for example, allows cell motion and change of form.

Cis - verses *trans*- fatty acids

Essential fatty acids are arguably the key molecules in the body. Because of their special structural patterns and electromagnetic characteristics, they form part of every intercellular messenger and communicator molecule, and every cellular membrane in the living body. Without them, the proteins and DNA molecules, which have created such scientific excitement in the past, would not be able to function. If the delicate – and very specifically located – double bonds in their structure are altered in any way, the biological activity of the essential fatty acid is lost. Therefore, it is important to consider the difference between *cis*- and *trans*- fatty acids.

These terms describe how atoms are arranged within a molecule. The same substance, with the same chemical composition, can exist in several structural arrangements, called *isomers*. Isomers of the same molecule do not have the same biological activity.

Concerning fatty acid activity, *cis*- and *trans*- isomers are important. In the *cis*- form, two functional, or bio-active groups are located on the same side of the molecule. In the *trans*- form, the functional groups are on opposite sides of the molecule. In other words, in isomers of a specific fatty acid, the two functional groups are at the same point in the carbon chain, but face differently. In the *cis-* form, they sit beside one another; in the *trans-* form they mirror each other, on opposite sides of the chain. The point at which these differences occur is at the location of a double bond.

The differences between *cis-* and *trans-* forms can be considerable. As the general rule in fats, for example, the *cis-* forms remain liquid, while the *trans-* configurations are solid.

In terms of diet, it is well known that fatty acids from animal tissues are almost all saturated, and fats obtained from plants are almost all unsaturated, although the degree of unsaturation varies (monounsaturated verses polyunsaturated, for example). Naturally occurring unsaturated fatty acids have at least one *cis-* double bond in their structure, and these are the seats of their greatest biological activity. Without this *cis-*bond, the 'essential' nature of the fatty acid is lost.

The trouble begins when natural oils are altered from their normal *cis-* type to *trans*. The resulting molecular structures are not only unable to carry out the function of the original design; they actually compete with the *cis-*forms. Therefore, *trans-*fatty acids, like those produced when some margarine manufacturers harden polyunsaturated oils to make a more attractive product for the market, actually increase the amount of *cis-*essential fatty acids you should consume to meet your body's requirements.

A word about margarine: some products are very good sources of polyunsaturated fatty acids, while others are not. It all depends on the method used to produce a solid spread from liquid vegetable oils. During your next shopping trip, read the manufacturer's label. If you are holding a package containing hydrogenated, *trans-*fats, reach for another brand – or, consider using a small quantity of butter. Hydrogenated margarine and butter contain the same number of calories per unit of weight, and the body uses *trans-*polyunsaturated fats as if they are saturated fats, but the flavours are certainly different!

Notice that I have said *trans-*fats increase your need for *cis-* forms of fatty acids. I have not said, as has been reported in some sectors of the popular media, that *trans-* fatty acids increase the risk of coronary heart disease. It is true, however, regarding blood cholesterol, as *trans-*fats act like the saturated fats they are intended to replace, and studies show that both increase cholesterol levels. On the other hand, repeated experiments show that *cis*-isomers of fatty acids lower chol-esterol levels. Writing in *Nutrition Reviews*, in 1993, Dr Thomas H. Applewhite pointed out that future experiments on this topic should evaluate the effects of *trans*-isomers in the presence of controlled amounts of *cis*-fatty acids. This is an important clue about how scientists are beginning to see the competitive relationship between saturated, *trans*-fats, and *cis*-forms of essential fatty acids.

Essential fatty acids and cell membranes

Essential fatty acids probably have their most important influence as components of cellular membranes. Each cell in the body is not only wrapped in a flexible covering two molecules thick, it is powered by a complex of sub-cellular particles – the organelles which I mentioned earlier – which are also made up of these thin layers. Essential fatty acids are important structural components of all membranes, whether they are inside or surround a cell, and their concentration in cell membranes can be measured. To describe the quality and quantity of essential fatty acids in membranes, scientists have defined a number known as the *Unsaturation Index*, which describes the total amount of essential fatty acids in a known quantity of membrane multiplied by the number of double bonds in the essential fatty acid identified. The Unsaturation Index has been shown to influence both their *fluidity* and *flexibility*. But, what do these terms mean?

When discussing cell membranes, 'fluidity' and 'flexibility' refer to the capacity of cell membranes to allow the easy flow of molecules through them, and to bend and move in their environment. As an example, a red blood cell is a round, flat object that, under a microscope, appears to have a consistent ridged form when compared with the flowing, irregular shapes of white blood cells. But, to be effective, both types of cells need to bend and change shape in order to move within the body. The various types of blood cells move in and out between the single cell linings of blood capillaries, and roam the body tissues when necessary. Under normal conditions, red blood cells remain flowing within the arteries and veins of the body's vascular system. However, they, too, require flexibility.

The specific activity of red blood cells is to carry oxygen supplies to tissue cells, and remove waste carbon dioxide. These transfers take place in the smallest tubes of the vascular system – the capillaries. Anyone having watched red blood cells flow through the tiny capillaries in skin will know that red cells seem to stack up and then squeeze as the pressure of the flow of plasma behind them forces them into and through the thin lumen of these blood vessels. To squeeze through the capillaries, the membrane structure of red cells must be pliable enough to allow modification in their shape. Research has shown that this 'fluidity' depends on the amount of essential fatty acids in the membrane.

Red blood cells which are low in essential fatty acid, are 'stiff', and appear to increase the thickness of blood, which in turn has been shown to decrease its ability to carry oxygen to tissue cells. Blood viscosity has been clinically linked with heart disease. Other research indicates that white blood cells, important players in an inflammatory response, are also less active when essential fatty acid tissue levels are low.

The decreased flexibility of blood cells which leads to an impaired capacity to function has been linked with various illnesses and diseases. These are discussed in some detail later.

The precise form of the essential fatty acids incorporated into membranes appears to control aspects of their function. Omega-3 fatty acids should be mentioned here, because there is considerable interest in their nutritional value, particularly as it pertains to heart disease. Although the omega-3 essential fatty acids may have as many – or more – double bonds as those classified as omega-6 series, they are unable to reverse the effects of essential fatty acid deficiency on cell membranes.

But the importance of membrane essential fatty acids goes far beyond structural behaviour of cells; they also influence the behaviour and function of proteins, the other major component of membranes. Protein molecules are critical to key biological activities, and their physical positions and environment must be biologically accurate for them to function. It is clinically significant that changes in the level of unsaturation in the lipid 'sea' in which proteins 'swim' influences their ability to interact with other molecules.

Essential fatty acids in cell communicators

Essential fatty acids are the primary element in the small, short-lived molecules acting as communicators between body cells. Pause for a moment to think about the staggering sum of individual cells in the body, and the many types of information that must be conveyed between them to maintain the normal chain of biological activity that makes up the processes of life. Such insight provides some idea of the vastness of this topic and its implications for medical research. Three specific types of molecules in which essential fatty acids are particularly important are: gamma-linolenic acid, the first metabolic product formed from linoleic acid, and two metabolites of gamma-linolenic acid, prostaglandin E1 (PGE1) and 15-OH-DGLA.

Prostaglandins: the basics

Obviously, many hundreds of scientists, besides those mentioned thus far in this book, have contributed to our understanding of the roles essential fatty acids play in human health and disease. One other important name in the history of fatty acid research is von Euler, a Swedish research chemist. In the 1930s von Euler identified a new, highly active form of molecule in semen. Thinking that these molecules were produced by the prostate gland, he gave them the misnomer, prostaglandins.

Prostaglandins produce a wide range of reactions in the body. Some activities attributed to a particular family of prostaglandins, the PGE1 series, which are derived from gamma-linolenic acid, are:

• inhibit abnormal cell proliferation;
• lower arterial pressure;
• inhibit cholesterol synthesis;
• inhibit inflammation; and
• activate certain white blood cells.

Not all the effects of prostaglandins are pleasant, however, and another group of these substances, known as PGE2 series, actually increase pain and inflammation. However, on the positive side of the balance sheet, they help stimulate the uterus and protect against peptic ulcers. Like members of the PGE1 series, some of these substances have been produced synthetically for pharmaceutical purposes. For example, *Gemepost* has been developed to soften and dilate the cervix. *Alprostadil,* a synthetic form of PGE1, is used to help in certain types of cardiac surgical procedures on infants.

Prostaglandins are one of several types of highly interactive, short-lived, molecules derived from essential fatty acids. Others are so-called eicosanoids and leukotrienes. These substances are the second-by-second regulators of most tissue activities in the body, and vital to tissue equilibrium. Again, if the diet is deficient in the parent essential fatty acid from which these hormone-like substances are derived, or if their conversion is blocked in any way, normal tissue activity is altered. Over the long-term, degenerative illnesses will result.

Controlling cholesterol

Research has established two ways in which essential fatty acids control cholesterol. First, PGE1 and other metabolites of gamma-linolenic acid inhibit cholesterol synthesis and aid in its transport across cell membranes. These biological activities have important medical implications.

Second, essential fatty acids aid the transport of cholesterol. To be moved around the body, whether to be used in a biological process or stored, cholesterol must be linked, or esterified with a fatty acid. The fatty acid's degree of saturation decides the solubility of the resulting 'ester', and therefore the ease of its movement in the watery environment of blood plasma and intercellular fluids. For example, cholesterol esters containing saturated fatty acids are less soluble than those formed with monounsaturates; and monounsaturated fatty acids produce esters less soluble than polyunsaturated fatty acids.

Essential fatty acids and skin permeability

The fourth major role identified for essential fatty acids is their ability to maintain the skin's impermeability to water. Research studies show that, in the absence of omega-6 fatty acids, skin loses its ability to shed water. According to Dr David Horrobin, it loses its 'waterproofing'. Normal protection returns when linoleic acid and gamma-linolenic acid are administered. As this is not true with other essential fatty acids, the specific molecular structure of these substances must be a critical factor.

Skin is not the only body tissue that controls the flow of fluids. The blood-brain barrier and tissues lining the gastro-intestinal tract also selectively decide the molecules that pass through them. For example, the brain is encased in a thin layer of lining cells, called endothelium, which controls the types of molecules allowed to pass from the blood into the tissues of the brain. This is a very new area of research, and much remains to be learned about the role fatty acids play in selecting and rejecting ions and molecules allowed to cross tissue frontiers. Nonetheless, it is difficult to avoid postulating about the possible relationships between essential fatty acid deficiency and illness.

The complicated families of essential fatty acid

To recap: there are two families of essential fatty acids – the omega-6 and the omega-3. Plants and plant seeds are good sources of the omega-6 variety, and while we frequently associate the omega-3 series with fish oil, it is, in fact, also a product of certain plants, such as grasses and water vegetation. When fish and other animals feed on these plants, omega-3 fatty acids are stored in their oil or fat deposits.

Omega-6 and omega-3 fatty acids: their structures compared

Counting from the methyl end of the carbon chain, the first point of unsaturation in an omega-3 fatty acid occurs after the third carbon. In an omega-6 molecule, it occurs after the sixth carbon. This difference in the location of the first unsaturated link between carbon atoms greatly affects the biological activity of molecules. So, it is wrong to think that omega-3 and omega-6 essential fatty acids can be substituted for one another in their therapeutic and biological importance. (The reason why the count starts at the methyl group end, or tail end, of the carbon chain of a fatty acid is that the methyl group remains unchanged even after the fatty acid has been transformed by the addition of two or more carbon atoms to the 'clasp' end of the chain, as it is the methyl group end which determines much of the molecule's biological activity.)

The scientific names, or nomenclature, define much more about the structure of the fatty acid. For example, the nomenclature for gamma-linolenic acid is 18:3n-6. This tells us that there are 18 carbons in its chain, that it has three unsaturated links between carbon atoms, and that the first point of unsaturation follows the sixth carbon in its chain. Arachidonic acid, another important essential fatty acid, is 20:4n-6. Among other things, the names of these essential fatty acids tell us they are from the same family of molecules.

To be even more precise, the full descriptive nomenclature for a fatty acid molecule defines exactly where all the points of unsaturation are found. For example, gamma-linolenic acid is (delta) 6,9,12:18:3(n-6). Points of unsaturation fall after the sixth, ninth, and twelfth carbon atoms in a chain of 18 carbon atoms.

In the body, fatty acids are found both floating free and linked to other molecules. When linked with other structures, fatty acids become known as esters, and the process is known as 'esterification'. Free floating fatty acids are, therefore, referred to as 'unesterified'. When a fatty acid is 'esterified', it looses its 'clasp', or carboxyl group, and hooks on to another molecule with the resulting 'hook', or valence. The esterification may be with a much larger, round and powerful cholesterol; or be joined to a molecule of glycerol. Energy stored in the body as fat takes the form of 'triglyceride', which is nothing more sinister that a molecule of glycerol esterified with three fatty acid molecules.

One reason why the location of a molecule's points of unsaturation is important is that each unsaturated link in the chain gives it a bend, and changes its shape. The molecule's 'bends' give shape and form to other molecules, and to larger structures; for example, they contribute to the fluidity and flexibility of cell membranes. If the bends are in the wrong places, the molecule cannot fulfil its necessary biological functions.

There is much to be learned about the structure of fatty acids and their biological activity. We do know now, however, that the structure of fatty acid molecules – and particularly the essential fatty acids – influence the structure and biological capacity of the cell membranes they help form, and contribute to the activity of the many specialized molecules into which essential fatty acids are incorporated.

How much essential fatty acid do humans require?

Based on animal studies, it has been estimated that between 1 and 2 per cent of total calories consumed should be from linoleic acid – like that found in safflower oil. Smaller amounts should be provided by fatty acids derived from linoleic, including gamma-linolenic acid and arachidonic acid.

Let us do some extrapolations: linoleic, gamma-linolenic, and arachidonic acids should provide approximately 1.5 per cent of the total calories in our diet. If a person is of normal size and physically active, he or she may consume on average 2,500 cal-ories a day; 1.5 per cent of that is approximately 38 calories. Since one gram of fat is equivalent to 9 calories, those 38 cal-ories equal 4.2 grams of omega-6 fatty acids a day. These calculations agree with advice from most experts, who consider 5 grams daily of essential fatty acids necessary for average adults.

It is very important to note that *this baseline amount of 5 grams a day is for essential fatty acids only, and not for total fat.* It also represents an estimate of requirements in a fit person; not one who is on a diet, pregnant, ill, or subjecting their body to insult from cigarette smoke or excessive amounts of alcohol. Many diet experts go astray on this point, and recommend daily fat levels that are far too low. Some exercise and diet gurus seem to have confused those 5 grams of essential fatty acids we require with our total requirement for fats. Over a long period of dieting, that may result in borderline deficiency symptoms.

But westerners eat so much fat – how can we be deficient in any one kind?

It is true that, over the past few decades, total fat content in the normal western diet has increased, and this increase includes the amount of essential fatty acids. Estimates of linoleic acid in the normal American diet today are in the region of 10-20g per day. Surely this is enough to ward off any deficiency problems, you may think.

Well, things are not that simple. To begin with, the average diet is also loaded with saturated fats, and as higher levels of saturates increase the need for unsaturates, this may be one explanation for an increase in degenerative diseases now being linked with essential fatty acid deficiency. Hidden saturated fats in burgers and ice cream may blank out benefits from the olive oil in the salad dressing.

Next, there is the problem of processed food. This takes us back to the discussion of *cis-* and *trans-* fatty acids. Some experts believe that the total daily intake of abnormal *trans*-fats in a typical western diet may be as high as 6-12g a day. Recall that these *trans*-fats are 'deactivated' essential fatty acids; that accounts for a large proportion of what we think we are ingesting as linoleic acid and its metabolites. Also, *trans-* fats compete with normal *cis-* fatty acids, thus increasing their requirement in most cases.

In conclusion: the western diet enjoyed in the United States, the United Kingdom, and much of the rest of the western world may simply not contain sufficient quantities of *cis-*, or *active*, essential fatty acids.

So, what happens then?

There may not be enough fatty acids to meet normal body needs, particularly as there are circumstances which block the conversion of linoleic acid into gamma-linolenic acid (*see Figure 5*). This results in what experts call a 'relative' essential fatty acid deficiency. An important substance is available to the body in levels so low as to slowly cause physical problems, but the system as a whole keeps ticking over.

Consider again the chart of metabolic derivatives from omega-6 and omega-3 fatty acids (*see Figure 3*). The foods we eat

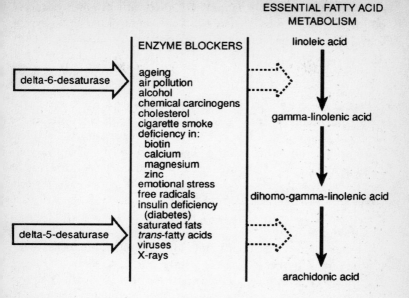

Figure 5 Lifestyle factors which interfere with our linoleic acid conversion process

supply most of our omega-6 fatty acids in the form of linoleic acid. Many of the conditions that destroy the effectiveness of linoleic acid do so by blocking conversion to gamma-linolenic acid (*see Figure 5*). That is why supplementation with oils rich in gamma-linolenic acid get around many of the problems caused by smoking, high levels of foods rich in saturated fats, excessive alcohol, some viral infection, and so on. Even normal ageing takes its toll on the amount of benefit you receive from the *cis*-essential fatty acids in your diet.

Omega-6 and omega-3 fatty acids: is there a difference?

As I have said before, some people have the idea that omega-3 and omega-6 fatty acids are the same; and still others believe the omega-3 fatty acids are the more important essential fatty acids. Neither is the case. I recently suggested to a friend that she should consider supplementing her diet with evening primrose oil for several months, to see if it would control her PMS symptoms. She explained this was not necessary, because she already took a daily dose of omega-3-rich fish oil. We had a cup of tea, and talked through some basic concepts concerning competition and differences in the world of essential fatty acids.

Part of the confusion about the relative value of various unsaturated oils stems from overly enthusiastic reports in the press about fish oil and the low risk of heart disease among Eskimos. This population survives on a diet dominated by fat, and containing almost no plant materials. Because one of the major components of the Eskimo diet is oily fish, some investigators concluded the link between diet and a low risk of heart disease was fish oil: the omega-3 fatty acids had a protective effect, it was thought.

At this point, we should note that investigators believe the omega-3 and omega-6 fatty acids are metabolized by the same sequence of enzymes. This sequence begins with delta-6-desaturase. What is more, this enzyme sequence appears to competitively favour the omega-3 fatty acids. When the omega-3 and omega-6 fats are combined in the same laboratory experiments, competition by the omega-3 fatty acids inhibits metabolism of the omega-6 molecules. This appears to block the formation of some substances that increase inflammation, and may be one reason why fish oil has been demonstrated to help many patients suffering from rheumatoid arthritis.

While this competition may theoretically have some benefits – such as a possible blocking of essential fatty acid metabolites that stimulate inflammation – there also appear to be more sinister consequences. Evidence from scientific investigations strongly suggests that the administration of fish oils may actually have negative effects; raising blood levels of LDL-cholesterol and inhibiting kidney function. As LDL-cholesterol levels have been shown to reflect the level of risk from coronary heart disease, these findings would suggest that omega-3 fatty acids do not have the protective influence on the cardiovascular system suggested by some epidemiologists.

So, what about the Eskimos? It seems that Eskimos enjoy interesting differences in the way their bodies metabolize fats. They seem to have at least one slight variation in the all-important fatty acid enzyme sequence. Perhaps, it has been suggested, they have no delta-5 desaturase; or, if they do possess this enzyme, it reacts more slowly than in non-Eskimo populations. Whatever the case, the important thing is that – whether eating a native or western diet – Eskimos appear to have elevated levels of dihomo-gamma-linolenic acid, and low levels of arachidonic acid. This pattern of fatty acids appears to have great health advantages for the cardiovascular system.

What happens when fish oil alone is administered to westerners? The ratios of dihomo-gamma-linolenic acid and arachidonic acid are opposite to those observed in the Eskimos. The westerners' levels of dihomo-gamma-linolenic acid falls precipitately, probably because of the inhibition of conversion from linoleic acid to gamma-linolenic acid resulting from competition by the omega-3 fatty acids.

In that case, what can be done to make westerners more like Eskimos? Offer a blend of oils: fish oil with a second oil which contains a high proportion of gamma-linolenic acid – evening primrose oil would be a good choice. The answer appears to rest in the fact that, while the omega-3 fatty acids block conversion of linoleic acid to gamma-linolenic acid, and dihomo-gamma-linolenic acid to arachidonic acid, they do not appear to affect the conversion of gamma-linolenic acid to dihomo-gamma-linolenic acid. By administering adequate doses of gamma-linolenic acid along with the fish oil, there is no drop in dihomo-gamma-linolenic acid, but the production of arachidonic acid from dihomo-gamma-linolenic acid is blocked. This results in a fatty acid pattern similar to that normally found in Eskimos.

This is not to suggest that omega-3 fatty acids do not have important biological functions, only that they are more limited than publicity about them would lead us to believe.

Omega-6 EFAs more biologically important than omega-3

There are several arguments supporting this claim, but what other evidence is there to support it? First, please give a thought to zebras. Like other members of the genus *Equus*, zebras eat almost nothing but grass. Grass is an interesting plant. It contains omega-6 fatty acids, but by far its highest percentage of fatty acids are of the omega-3 variety – primarily alpha-linolenic acid. However, when scientists conduct an analysis of fatty tissue from a zebra, they find that the dominant essential fatty acids are from the omega-6 series. This can only be interpreted as an indication that zebras and similar animals selectively store omega-6 essential fatty acids over omega-3 acids, despite their dietary levels.

When tissues from animals fed their normal diets are tested to determine the ratio of omega-6 to omega-3 fatty acids they contain, the range lies between 3:1 to 9:1. This is true for meat-eaters and grass-eaters alike.

Second, the literature on fats and nutrition contain numerous reports stating that animals, placed on experimental diets containing absolutely no omega-6 fatty acids, will develop obvious biochemical and biological abnormalities in every major organ group in their bodies. The opposite is true for animals placed on a diet lacking omega-3 essential fatty acids: and only the most recent, highly sophisticated investigative techniques demonstrate abnormalities in brain and retinal function.

And third, if experimental animals are kept on diets lacking all omega-6 and omega-3 fatty acids long enough for deficiency symptoms to appear, treatment with omega-6 essential fatty acids will quickly reverse signs of tissue degeneration. The same reversal will not occur if the animals are treated with omega-3 essential fatty acids. In fact, some symptoms of deficiency may become worse, particularly those involving the skin and capillaries.

Why the omega-6 essential fatty acids are important

Research links essential fatty acid deficiency with a number of diseases, and cancer, cardiovascular disease, inflammation and auto-immune disorders, breast pain, premenstrual syndrome, skin disorders, osteoporosis, multiple sclerosis, and diabetic complications are among them. Taken at face value, these facts are very reassuring to the casual observer; something as straightforward and understandable as a nutritional deficiency appears to have a causal link with some of the most devastating physical conditions and illnesses in modern society. On closer inspection, however, that same casual observer will stop and ask, how can this be so? How can all these complex diseases be related to something as simple as low intake levels of specific fats common in most of the foods we eat? How can essential fatty acids be involved in illnesses as different in characteristics and symptoms as breast pain and bone degeneration? And, what are we doing to medically combat these conditions?

chapter four

THE HEALTH CONNECTION

WHAT happens when not enough essential fatty acids are available to meet the body's requirements? Over the long term, a form of marginal malnutrition, or borderline deficiency, develops which can cause changes in cell membrane structures, in the transport of cholesterol, and in the communication systems between cells. Depending on the extent of this nutritional deficiency, and any pre-existing medical conditions, the groundwork is laid for the development of one or more degenerative illnesses.

Considering the complexity of the subject, the confused and conflicting advice given to the public is not surprising. Scientists are just beginning to unravel the complicated effects of these changes on our health status. Nonetheless, it is possible to guess at certain types of medical consequences.

A growing body of international research is demonstrating the value of treating certain medical conditions with food supplements containing essential fatty acids. Thus far, results for a number of illnesses are very exciting. But even more impressive are results from the clinical trials of a new family of drugs produced from essential fatty acids. These promise hope for patients with a range of diseases such as cancer, rheumatoid arthritis, and diabetes. There follows some highlights of progress being made in targeting the effects of essential fatty acids on normal growth and health, as well as specific clinical conditions.

Healthy babies

Gamma-linolenic acid, alpha-linolenic acid and their metabolites are vital to good health and normal growth during infancy and childhood. From the beginning of life in the embryo – rapid development and the flow of information between cells require a balanced and adequate supply of essential fatty acids. They are fundamental.

This raises an important issue in the bottle-versus-breast feeding debate. A fully breast-fed baby gets everything it needs from its mother's milk during the early, critical stages of growth; including all of the essential vitamins and proteins, minerals, carbohydrates – and – essential fatty acids.

Human milk is rich in both omega-6 and omega-3 essential fatty acids. When compared with pasteurized cows' milk, mature human milk contains five times more polyunsaturated and almost 50 per cent more monounsaturated fats. Besides the primary forms of essential fatty acids, linoleic and alpha-linolenic acids, metabolites of these molecules are also present. Analysis shows human milk contains gamma-linolenic acid, dihomo-gamma-linolenic, arachidonic acid and, from the omega-3 series, eicosapentaenoic acid (EPA) and docosahexaenoic acid (DHA). Some scientists believe these substances are present in mothers' milk because the enzyme system needed to metabolize fatty acids is not fully formed in the very young child.

There is a difference between breast and bottle-fed infants. Studies show bottle fed babies consistently have lower levels of omega-6- unsaturated essential fatty acids in their blood than breast-fed infants. Most formulae are not fortified with essential fatty acids. Some contain linoleic acid and sometimes alpha-linolenic acid, but only a few products contain metabolites of these essential fatty acids. In Japan, Snow Brand, which is fed to approximately 30 per cent of Japanese formula-fed infants, contains evening primrose oil to supplement the diet with gamma-linolenic acid. Farley's milk for young infants, supplied in the United Kingdom, is another example of a milk formula supplemented with gamma-linolenic acid. At the time of writing, these cases are more the exception than the rule. When choosing an infant formula, look at the list of ingredients and make sure it contains essential fatty acids. And remember how fragile these substances are; follow sell-by dates, and keep unused products in a cool place.

Essential fatty acids for the elderly

As the human body ages, it loses its capacity to convert essential fatty acids into their more biologically active derivatives. Specifically, ageing affects the activity of the enzyme, delta-6-desaturase. Failure of this enzyme creates a deficiency of fatty acids within both the omega-6 and omega-3 series. Low supplies of these substances speed the ageing process and add to the possibility of developing a number of degenerative illnesses, including heart disease.

Experts suggest food supplements containing metabolites of linoleic and alpha-linolenic acid help fill the shortfall in fatty acid metabolites. By filling this gap, signs of old age can be delayed, and certain illnesses prevented or slowed.

Coronary heart disease

Coronary artery and heart disease are major killers in western society. Although billions have been spent on research into its cause, the answer remains unclear. Smoking, high blood fat levels, stress, and too much saturated fat in the diet have all been statistically linked to high rates of the disease. From this list, two things are evident. First, a list of the factors most closely associated with heart disease are very similar to a list of factors that destroy the enzyme, delta-6-dehydrogenase; and second, fat is somehow a part of the origins of cardiovascular illness.

Decades have past since Hugh Sinclair first identified the possibility that coronary heart disease might be caused by inadequate amounts of omega-6 fatty acids in the system. More recently, examination of the true picture of coronary heart disease suggests a role for omega-3 fatty acids as well. Omega-3 fatty acids are particularly effective in lowering blood triglycerides, which is not true of their omega-6 cousins. Results from clinical trials with linoleic acid, and evidence from observations concerning the surprising low rate of coronary disease among the Eskimos, suggest an important protective role for dietary supplements containing both a source rich in gamma-linolenic acid, such as evening primrose oil or linseed oil, and fish oil.

The reasons why people living in western societies develop

heart disease are unclear, but five medical conditions are usually associated with increased risk from heart disease:

- Elevated cholesterol levels
- Elevated triglyceride levels
- Hypertension
- An increased tendency for blood platelets to stick together
- Diabetes

On careful study of the research done to date, evidence of a direct link between cardiovascular disease and individual factors in this list is weak, and very difficult to assess outside very large population studies. Perhaps surprisingly, in the light of media emphasis on the other risk factors, statistical analysis shows the closest link exists between diabetes and heart disease. Diabetics suffering from one or more of the other coronary risk factors are most likely to die of heart disease.

But, research by the Efamol Research Institute, has identified another factor strongly associated with an increased risk of coronary disease, and that is low intake and low tissue levels of linoleic acid. Somehow, until recently, this fact has not been given much attention by the medical community or the media.

It may be that the level of linoleic acid metabolites is more important than the primary essential fatty acid itself, because research shows that low concentrations of both dihomo-gamma-linolenic and arachidonic acid in blood and body fat are stronger indicators of risk from coronary disease than levels of linoleic acid alone. These low concentrations may arise if the body is unable to desaturate linoleic acid.

This theory has been tested by feeding large amounts of safflower oil (a rich source of linoleic acid) to men at risk from coronary heart disease. After a period, changes in their body fats were compared with samples obtained from men fed equal quantities of evening primrose oil, which contains like amounts of linoleic acid, but with the addition of gamma-linolenic acid. Tissue from the group fed safflower oil had increased levels of linoleic acid, but there was no effect on the deposition of its metabolites. By contrast, the group fed evening primrose oil had significant rises in their levels of linoleic acid metabolites as well, especially dihomo-gamma-linolenic acids, which has a strong association with lessened risk of heart disease.

These findings strongly suggest that people at risk from coronary heart disease do not have a normal capacity to metabolize linoleic acid into its derivatives. As these derivatives are necessary in controlling high blood-cholesterol and triglyceride levels, and platelet aggregation, a block in the conversion of linoleic to gamma-linolenic acid may be the real cause of heart disease. This block may be because of an inbuilt metabolic problem, or because of some extraneous cause: smoking, excessive amounts of saturated fat, increasing age, stress, and so on – all expand the body's demand for dietary gamma-linolenic acid. It is a block that can be bypassed by the administration of evening primrose oil and other sources of gamma-linolenic acid.

Rheumatoid arthritis and other inflammatory diseases

Rheumatoid arthritis is a degenerative disease of the joints, although other connective tissue may also be affected. In some people, the disease begins and remains in a relatively mild state for years; in others, it destroys their pattern of life.

Rheumatoid arthritis is an *autoimmune disease* in which the body is attacked by its own immune system, and should not be confused with osteoarthritis, which involves degeneration of the cartilage tissues lining the joints.

The explanation of the cause of rheumatoid arthritis is still debated by scientific experts, but apparently something goes wrong with the body's balance of the various types of prostaglandins: those minute intercellular messengers that control much of what happens in the fluid-filled space between cells. Recall from the previous chapter that there are two primary forms of prostaglandins: PGE1, which suppresses inflammation and excessive immune reactions in tissues, and the PGE2 series that causes inflammation.

In rheumatoid arthritis, PGE1 levels drop and the PGE2 series becomes dominant, especially in bone and its surrounding connective tissue. Current medical practice is to suppress the PGE2s, and the inflammation that results from their activity, by treatment with nonsteroidal anti-inflammatory drugs (NSAIDs)

– for example, ibuprofen, certain drugs based on cortisone, gold and penicillamine. All these have varying levels of success, and all have side-effects. Taken in excess, NSAIDs can cause abdominal pain, heartburn and even gastric bleeding. None of these forms of therapy permanently alters the imbalance of prostaglandins at the root of the problem.

Hope for new methods of treatment for rheumatoid arthritis seems to rest on some form of intervention involving essential fatty acids. Help is expected to come from new drugs, but that is some way in the distance. For now, the way to help patients – particularly in the early stages of the condition – is by using dietary supplements containing both omega-6 and omega-3 fatty acids. Experiments on humans hold out great hope, and good results have been achieved using a blend of evening primrose and fish oil. Tested over a period of months, patients given this combination have reported striking results. In placebo-controlled studies 90 per cent of patients reported feeling better after taking the essential fatty acid mixture, as opposed to 30 per cent who were given the non-therapeutic placebo. And, there is good evidence patients treated with essential fatty acids require fewer NSAIDs to control their symptoms, thereby reducing any possible side-effects from these drugs.

Cancer

In December 1994, Scotia Pharmaceuticals Plc announced the final stages of clinical trails for a successful cancer treatment based on a lithium salt of gamma-linolenic acid, EF13. After years of careful investigation, EF13 has been shown to have significant value in treating patients with pancreatic cancer, and several other forms of this disease. Pancreatic cancer is a most cataclysmic form of malignant tumour, and most patients are beyond surgical help at the time of diagnosis. Intensive chemotherapy can only extend their lives for a short period. The effects of the therapy are usually such that both patients and doctors frequently opt instead for palliative care to alleviate pain and control symptoms until death. Under these conditions, EF13 is particularly significant, because tests showed it to be a more effective means of extending life than highly toxic chemotherapy, and with none of the common side effects of nausea and vomiting, hair loss, extreme fatigue, and suppression of the immune system. Many patients treated with the new compound reported an improved sense of well-being, and some experienced weight gain: an unusual circumstance in cases of pancreatic cancer. Tests are going on with patients suffering from malignant melanoma, breast, colon, brain, and kidney cancer.

Scotia's early findings leading up to the development of EF13 were first announced in the early 1980s, and have since been confirmed in independent laboratories around the world, including ones at the National Cancer Institute of the USA, the University of Kyoto, The University of Western Ontario, Yale University, the University of Hyderabad, and University College Hospital, London. Many investigators look to these developments as the first in a series of gentler, more effective cancer drugs.

EF13 grew from early laboratory observation that gamma-linolenic acid and its derivative, dihomo-gamma-linolenic acid, kills cancer cells without harming normal cells. To date, this phenomenon has been successfully shown in several different types of cancer cells.

However, considerable confusion exists surrounding the question of foods containing polyunsaturated fats and the incidence of cancer. Recent media stories have linked vegetable oils, linoleic acid and its metabolites, with an increased risk of breast cancer, but there are good grounds for questioning the research on which these press reports are based.

First, the research was done on rats, not humans. According to David Horrobin, writing in the professional publication *Progress in Lipid Research*, 'The main problem [with these studies] is that evening primrose oil, containing gamma-linolenic acid, should on this hypothesis enhance the risk of mammary cancer even more than the linoleic acid-containing vegetable oils. Instead, evening primrose oil consistently inhibits cancer growth and development when fed to animals. This effect of primrose oil is consistent with human rather than animal studies of cancer. No human study has ever shown vegetable fats in general or linoleic acid in particular to be associated with cancer risk. Moreover, a high intake of linoleic acid was associated with a reduced risk of metastasis [transfer of a disease to other parts of the body]. High levels of linoleic acid and its metabolites in actual human cancers were associated with a more favourable prognosis. Thus, in humans, and in animals, all the evidence is consistent with the idea that, whatever may be the effects of linoleic acid, the effects of gamma-linolenic acid and further metabolites are inhibitory to cancer growth.'

Osteoporosis

In the United Kingdom, one out of every five hospital beds is occupied by patients suffering from osteoporosis-related fractures. The combined number of women dying in the United Kingdom from breast, cervical and uterine cancer is less than the number dying from complications following hip fracture.

Osteoporosis is a debilitating disease, caused by the escape of calcium salts from bone, which affects both men and women; although post-menopausal women are, by far, at greater risk. To begin to understand this degenerative condition, think back to the earlier discussion of cells, and the mineral and protein deposits, or matrix, that surround pockets of cells in healthy cartilage and bone. When the conditions that control the balance of that matrix change, and its composition is altered, the strength and characteristics of the bone or cartilage are also changed. In bone, these changes cause a loss of calcium in the inter-cellular matrix, leading to a thinning and fragility of its structure.

Scientists disagree about the major cause of osteoporosis, although most admit the simple process of ageing is responsible for bone calcium loss. Other reasons given include inadequate quantities of calcium in the diet, and hormone imbalance. Matters are made worse by smoking and excessive intake of alcohol.

However, according to experts in the field, one of the major causes of osteoporosis is the failure of the gut to fully absorb calcium from the foods in our diet. This failure probably arises from deficiencies in the quantity of essential fatty acids present, because certain metabolites of both omega-6 and omega-3 fatty acids have been shown to help control the calcium absorption process. In addition, these same essential fatty acid metabolites are perceived by many experts as critical in controlling the amount of calcium excreted by the kidneys. If the essential fatty acids present are too few, or if their metabolism is blocked by a failure of the delta-6 desaturase enzyme, there is a risk of calcium deposits forming in the kidneys, and calcium leaking away from the bone.

Hormone replacement therapy (HRT) is one means doctors are using to control these conditions. However, this therapy has limitations. It can only be used by women; and, although bone calcium levels have been shown to fall after the age of 30, women cannot take HRT until menopause; and, older women who have not taken oestrogen hormones regularly from the time of their menopause, should not be treated with HRT.

Others scientists, seeking to better understand the biochemistry of osteoporosis, have established the importance of both gamma-linolenic acid and eicosapentaenoic acid in calcium metabolism and the maintenance of bone strength. Based on these findings, experts from Scotia Holdings have developed a system of prevention and treatment based on daily doses of calcium, gamma-linolenic acid, eicosapentaenoic acid and docosahexaenoic acid. This product appears to have no side-effects, even after long periods of use, and is suitable for all age-groups and both sexes.

PMS and mastalgia

In the early 1980s, the British courts reduced the sentences of two women convicted of murder to manslaughter because they were convinced each was suffering 'reduced responsibility' at the time of their crimes caused by severe symptoms of premenstrual syndrome (PMS). Unfortunately, although these dramatic findings hailed a more enlightened attitude towards PMS, over a decade later much remains to be done to help the millions of women who suffer each month.

Any woman suffering from PMS is familiar with its complex mix of physical and psychological characteristics. The combined effects of symptoms can range from a mild feeling of being unwell to severely debilitating conditions. For many women, PMS sets the schedule for their lives, and they plan major work and home activities around when they expect the next bout of discomfort and emotional upset to occur. Frequently, symptoms become worse as menstruation approaches, and then dissipate within 72 hours, or less, following the start of menstrual flow. Mood swings involving anxiety and depression, abdominal bloating, general water retention, food cravings and breast pain are all common characteristics of PMS that wreak havoc on personal relationships and on the ability to carry out day-to-day responsibilities.

Treating PMS is difficult because symptoms vary widely from one woman to the next; some may suffer more from mild water retention and bloating, while others may describe their primary complaint as the sudden occurrence of a 'black mood' that lasts for several days. Medical scientists have investigated many possible causes, including endocrine dysfunction and nutritional deficiencies, but none seems to provide an answer to the range of conditions reported by sufferers. As a result, doctors attitudes towards PMS vary; some are very supportive, while others offer little advice or help to their PMS patients. As a result, methods of treatment vary. Hormones – including progesterone – have been shown to help some patients. Diuretics and pain relief are useful means of controlling symptoms. And dietary changes have been shown to greatly effect some women. However, the most dramatic results have been achieved by the administration of dietary supplements of evening primrose oil – rich in gamma-linolenic acid.

There are good reasons to believe that high levels of saturated fat in the diet are linked with both breast pain and PMS. Many studies have shown abnormal patterns of blood and plasma fatty acids in breast pain sufferers. This may be owing to a failure in the normal metabolism of linoleic acid and an increased demand for one of its metabolites, arachadonic acid. As clinical research has shown that gamma-linolenic acid can relieve the symptoms of breast pain and PMT, a special gamma-linolenic acid compound, SP116 (*Efamast*), has been developed and licensed in the United Kingdom by the Department of Health.

Research has shown that in more than 70 per cent of women suffering from breast pain, the condition worsens before menstruation occurs; in others, there seems to be no connection between the two. An obvious hormonal connection exists between PMS and breast pain because both have been shown to be relieved by suppressing ovarian hormones, by either natural or medical means. However, research has not shown a clear relationship between abnormal levels of ovarian hormones and PMS. Nor has it been proved that there is a link between breast pain and levels of prolactin – the pituitary hormone that stimulates breast tissue. Both PMS and breast pain exist in the presence of normal levels of these hormones. Therefore, symptoms must be because of a condition that sensitizes tissues to their presence.

Research suggests the foods we eat, and the specific substances they include, are an important factor in controlling PMS and breast pain. These conditions are most common among women eating foods rich in fats – particularly saturated fats. Fats appear to be a key player in controlling the sensitivity of tissues to reproductive hormones, because clinical tests have demonstrated dramatic improvement in breast pain when the total level of dietary fat is greatly restricted.

Interestingly, many women who experience PMS also suffer from allergic – or atopic – skin disorders. Along with other symptoms, their skin conditions become worse some days prior to the start of their menstrual flow. Treatment with gamma-linolenic acid has been shown to improve both conditions.

Dietary fats may contribute to PMS and its related symptoms in three ways. First, cell membranes rich in saturated fatty acids attract and hold within the cell structure more molecules of steroid hormone than those rich in unsaturated fats, thereby exaggerating the effects of circulating hormones.

Second, steroid hormones – such as those produced by the ovaries – are attached to molecules of fatty acids while they are active in the body tissues. This linkage is called an 'ester'. Hormone esters containing saturated fats are more biologically active than those that involve unsaturated fatty acids.

The third possible connection between dietary fat and PMS involves the prostaglandins derived from the metabolites of gamma-linolenic acid. Specifically, prostaglandin PGE1 seems to reduce the biological activity of the pituitary hormone, prolactin, on peripheral tissues. If the materials needed to produce adequate amounts of PGE1 are limited, then normal circulating levels of prolactin can have an exaggerated effect. This effect may be especially pronounced in women with atopy (hypersensitivity), in whom the metabolic system is limited in its ability to form long-chain essential fatty acids. This could explain the link between PMS and certain other conditions. For example, some women with atopic eczema experience a severe worsening of their skin condition at the same time they suffer PMS symptoms. Irritable bowel syndrome (IBS) also increases in severity in many PMS suffers during the days leading up to their menstruation. Controlled studies have shown that both IBS and atopic eczema improve with evening primrose oil treatment in a significant number of cases, thus indicating a link between essential fatty acids and IBS.

It is important to remember that not all essential fatty acid studies have shown the same level of success in reducing or eliminating the symptoms of PMS, breast pain and irritable bowel syndrome. In part, this is because every patient presents unique characteristics related to age, diet, weight, metabolic activity and tissue composition. Because the chemical and biological interactions of body molecules are so complex and rapid, it is very difficult to know when the internal conditions are identical. What is more, not every study is conducted in the same way. Sometimes the differences between one experimental design and another are so obscure they are never recognized.

More important, in some circumstances, variation between the degrees of a treatment's success depends to some extent on the perceptions of the patient. In conditions as multifaceted as PMS, many factors are at work at any one time to influence the patient's judgement of her well-being. In cases of PMS, more so than in cyclical breast disease, a placebo effect may influence the patient's response to treatment. Consequently, despite the weight of evidence in favour of essential fatty acid treatment from PMS and breast pain, not all investigators are equally convinced of the value of essential fatty acids as a treatment.

Endometriosis

Endometriosis is another problem suffered by many women

during their childbearing years. Its origins are unknown, but its symptoms result from bits of endometrial tissue – the lining of the uterus – that break off and escape to other locations in the body, but usually in the pelvic cavity. These little pieces of tissue continue to respond to the cycle of female hormones, and each month they bleed, just as if they were still in the uterus. As there is no place for the blood to go, cysts often form around the patch of roving uterine tissue, and these may become as large as a small grapefruit. The symptoms of endometriosis vary, but can include abnormally heavy menstrual bleeding (the most common symptom), pain in the pelvis, back or abdomen, diarrhoea, constipation, painful defecation, and painful intercourse. (Endometriosis should not be confused with endometritis, which is caused by infection, and is also known as pelvic inflammatory disease.)

There is evidence that treatment with gamma-linolenic acid and eicosapentaenoic acid – an omega-3 fatty acid derived from alpha-linolenic acid – may help control the symptoms of endo-metriosis. This is probably because of the anti-inflammatory action of certain metabolites of these essential fatty acids, and because they could damp the peripheral effects of female steroid hormones without limiting their influence over reproductive tissues. Placebo-controlled studies of Scotia HGA, a complex of concentrated gamma-linolenic and eicosapentaenoic acids has demonstrated significant improvement in approximately 90 per cent of women.

Conditions involving the nervous system

Although the omega-6 fatty acids dominate, both omega-6 and omega-3 fatty acids are important in the formation of the complex network of billions of cells that make up the brain and central nervous system. By weight, about 60 per cent of the brain is fat – a greater percentage than in any other organ. Most of this fat is essential fatty acid.

If you stop to think about the brain in a developing child, you can see how important adequate amounts of essential fatty acids are, and why it is necessary to make certain very young children are not placed on very low fat diets. (In fact, children also need fat for energy and for general cell growth.)

Why do children living in societies where low-fat diets are the standard appear to develop normally? Again, the answer is complex. To begin with, children who appear to live on low-fat diets, for example children in the Far East and Africa, where vegetables and grains are the major source of nutrients, receive small but pure amounts of essential fatty acids every time they have a meal. Some come from the plants and fish, others are provided in the oil used in food preparation. Children fed this way are better served than children brought up on processed breakfast cereal and hot dogs.

Second, think about those hot dogs and sugary, highly processed breakfast cereal products. The form of a significant portion of unsaturated fatty acids contained in their original ingredients has probably changed from *cis-* to *trans-* acids by manufacturing processes. If the growing central nervous system cannot get all of the *cis-* fatty acids it needs for cell growth, it will manufacture some 'pseudo' polyunsaturated fatty acid, and where necessary, may use some *trans-*fats as well. We don't know what the results of these breaks with normal fatty acid structures are, but it is possible that these subtle differences in cells of the brain, spinal cord, the retinas of the eyes, and the peripheral nerves, have an effect on how our bodies function. They may affect the way people behave, and they may lay the foundation for certain disorders of the central nervous system.

For years, scientists have looked for connections between fatty acids and functions of the nervous system. While many important observations have been made, some of the most exciting were generated in an unexpected way. In the late 1980s, some very surprising evidence came from the World Health Organisation (WHO). A massive survey was undertaken in eight countries in Africa, the Americas, Asia and Europe to study the frequency and aftermath of schizophrenia. Under standard diagnostic methods and measures, investigators found that there was almost no variation in the occurrence of schizophrenia among the populations studied. However, there the similarities ended.

In some countries, schizophrenia was a serious, lifelong illness; in others, the disease was relatively mild and self-limiting. Statistical analyses were undertaken to explain these discrepancies. By far, the strongest correlation was with the fat content of the diet. The results were remarkable: there was a strong positive correlation between increased rates of schizophrenia and the presence of high levels of saturated fat in the diet. Conversely, there was a strong negative correlation between low rates of the disease and diets rich in vegetables, fruit and fish.

Very strong evidence suggested that essential fatty acids were involved in the evolution and continuation of whatever biological conditions are at the root of this disease. Studies in Japan, England, Ireland and the United States have shown a consistently low level of linoleic acid in blood samples taken from schizophrenic patients. Detailed studies of brain tissue show significant abnormalities in the fatty acids of the frontal lobes of schizophrenic patients.

This evidence led investigators to seek a medical breakthrough using some form of essential fatty acid product. The results have been mixed, but improvements in memory, and also several other symptoms, have been observed.

Other conditions involving the central nervous system and peripheral nerves have been linked with deficiencies or metabolic mistakes in the body's use of essential fatty acids. Some improvement has been observed in children with hyperkinesis, or hyperactivity. However, the way ahead for the therapeutic role essential fatty acids may play in this condition is unclear. Nor is it clear what role essential fatty acids play in the cause and control of multiple sclerosis; although the epidemiological evidence suggests that the disease is most prevalent in countries where the diet contains large amounts of saturated fats.

Where does this leave us? We know three things: human milk contains high levels of omega-6 and omega-3 metabolites, suggesting an innate need for these substances in growth and development. We know that the human brain is largely made up of fat, and that these are predominantly essential fatty acids. And we know that population studies suggest a positive correlation between saturated fat in the diet and certain diseases involving the central nervous system. From this, one can reasonably postulate that future therapeutic successes will come from developments involving essential fatty acids.

Alcohol and alcoholism

The relationship between alcohol (ethanol) and essential fatty acids is complex. One current nutritional theory suggests that small quantities of wine and spirits have a beneficial effect. It is claimed, for example, that red wine is good for the heart owing to some of its antioxidant properties. Simultaneously, other research shows us that alcohol drains the body's supply of essential fatty acids. It simultaneously depletes the amount of linoleic acid available from dietary sources, and increases the body's total demand for essential fatty acid metabolites. Thus, under the influence of alcohol the body's need for essential fatty acids escalates, but the usual sources are drained away in other directions.

For example, one way in which alcohol causes damage is by decreasing the amount of gamma-linolenic acid available for conversion into more biologically active metabolites. Alcohol inhibits the enzyme delta-6-desaturase and, in doing that, blocks the formation of linoleic acid into gamma-linolenic acid. This puts biological activities requiring gamma-linolenic acid and its further metabolites at risk. A heavy drinker at the dinner table may fill himself with foods rich in linoleic acid, but the alcohol in his system will make all or most of it useless by temporarily destroying the delicate biological systems needed for the creation of gamma-linolenic acid.

Alcohol has another damaging effect involving omega-6 fatty acids, further down the line of metabolic events. It blocks the transformation of dihomo-gamma-linolenic acid into the prostaglandin PGE1. PGE1 is an important 'tissue messenger'. Under normal circumstances, as stores of PGE1 are used and more is required, the need is met by the production of omega-6 metabolites from available linoleic acid. But, because alcohol hinders this chain of events by blocking delta-6-desaturase, another source of substrate must be found. As a result, precious body stores of dihomo-gamma-linolenic acid are quickly converted to PGE1, and exhausted. When this 'emergency' source of substrate is depleted, levels of PGE1 become dangerously low. As a result, the heavy drinker is open to risk from stroke, liver damage, heart attack, brain damage and infection.

Most people drink because it makes them feel good. That sense of euphoria probably results from a rush of PGE1 into the brain. Take a drink, increase your PGE1, and you will feel a warm glow of well-being. But watch out; a small amount of alcohol may improve your mood, but too much will deplete your PGE1 levels and leave you feeling very blue indeed! Unusually elevated quantities of PGE1 have been shown in blood taken from manic mental patients; the opposite is true in people suffering from clinical depression.

Pregnant women need to be particularly aware of the damage alcohol can inflict on their developing child. The reasons for this become clear when you consider the important functions essential fatty acids have in building normal cells and tissues, and the devastating effects alcohol has on the metabolism and utilization of omega-6 metabolites. It is reasonable that, if low levels of PGE1 can lead to liver disease, stroke and brain damage in an adult, they can seriously damage an unborn child.

Therapeutic regimes including gamma-linolenic acid and its metabolites have significant value in countering the physical effects of alcohol abuse. Controlled studies using gamma-linolenic acid on human subjects demonstrate success in managing the disastrous withdrawal symptoms experienced after the sudden denial of alcohol. Physical symptoms are relieved, liver function is rapidly improved, and fewer tranquillizers are needed to control extreme cases. Even more encouragingly for clinicians, patients who remain alcohol-free experience significant improvement in memory and motor-eye co-ordination.

Unfortunately, there is no evidence that omega-6 fatty acids can reduce the relapse rate of alcoholics.

Alzheimer's disease

The improved memory observed in alcoholic patients has stimulated interest in the possible benefits from essential fatty acids to people afflicted with Alzheimer's disease. Work by Horrobin and others clearly show Alzheimer's patients have major defects in tissue and blood essential fatty acids, suggesting a possible therapeutic role for essential fatty acids. The number of controlled studies testing this idea is still limited, but initial results suggest that products containing evening primrose oil, *Efamol* for example, have greater promise than most other therapies tested to date. In addition, the early work suggests that Alzheimer's disease may be related to excessive oxidation of essential fatty acids in brain tissue. The possible outcome may be a product combining essential fatty acids with some form of antioxidants.

Other medical conditions

Skin Disease: The link between essential fatty acids and good health is literally skin deep. Almost 50 years ago, in the laboratory where essential fatty acids were discovered, a technician noticed that the dermatitis on his hands improved when he increased the amount of linoleic acid he consumed. About the same time, scientists observing rats maintained on an essential fatty acid deficient diet saw they developed skin lesions closely resembling atopic eczema seen in humans.

Clinical research links atopic eczema with an inherited reduced rate of delta-6-desaturase activity. If this is the case, a therapeutic response should be obtained by treatment with omega-6 and omega-3 fatty acid metabolites. Remarkable success has been achieved in many patients by administering gamma-linolenic products, such as *Epogram*, with significant decreases in all symptoms, but especially itching. The exact mechanism for improvement is not clear, however, because not all patients experience improvement of their symptoms. Wider success has been achieved in early studies using a blend of evening primrose oil and fish oil.

Research has also shown essential fatty acids are important in managing more common skin conditions, such as acne and psoriasis.

Diabetic neuropathy: Over time, diabetic patients appear to lose their ability to desaturate essential fatty acids. This suggests that many secondary conditions associated with diabetes may be caused by their body tissues failing to receive adequate quantities of essential fatty acid metabolites. Two therapeutic strategies have been tested – one is to load these patients with linoleic acid, the master molecule of the omega-6 group; and the other is to directly supply metabolites from the omega-6 group.

Some considerable success has been achieved. In one large, six year study of non-insulin-dependent diabetics, those treated with diets containing four times the normal amount of linoleic acid developed far fewer complications involving the retina and cardiovascular system. Even more exciting results have been achieved in the treatment of diabetic neuropathy. During the progress of diabetes, peripheral nerve damage occurs which is thought to be caused by abnormal essential fatty acids in the structure of the neuronal membranes. A double-blind placebo-controlled study in humans has shown a reversal of diabetic neuropathy, which was possibly because of the replacement of damaged membrane molecules. These results point towards future control of this condition through diet and therapeutic products containing essential fatty acids and their derivatives.

Post-viral Fatigue Syndrome (ME): It is known that viral infections are characterized by reduced levels of linoleic acid, and by inhibition of delta-6 desaturase. Strong research evidence suggests that interferon, a substance necessary in the body's fight against viral infections, depends on both dihomo-gamma-linolenic and arachidonic acid to be effective. This suggests that essential fatty acids are important in controlling viral infections and their aftermath.

Applying this theory to practice has provided important insight into the treatment for patients suffering from post-viral fatigue syndrome, also known as myalgic encephalomyelitis (ME). Sixty patients were treated with *Efamol Marine* (80 per cent evening primrose oil and 20 per cent fish oil) for three months. To assess body levels of essential fatty acids, blood samples were taken and the fatty acid composition of red cell membranes analysed. These tests showed higher than normal levels of saturated and monounsaturated fatty acids, and reduced levels of both omega-3 and omega-6 fatty acids. At the beginning, midpoint and end of the study patients were evaluated for muscle weakness, pain, concentration level, perception of exhaustion, memory loss, vertigo, and depression. A control group – who did not receive *Efamol Marine* – were monitored using the same methods. In the end, the results were clear: symptoms improved in 85 per cent of the treated patients, but in only 17 per cent of the control patients. Red blood cell membranes from treated patients, tested at the conclusion of the study, contained normal levels of saturated, monounsaturated and omega-6 fatty acids, and slightly higher than normal levels of omega-3 derivatives.

Kidney disease: There are several reasons to believe continued research on the role of essential fatty acids and renal disease will prove fruitful. For example, the normal kidney is particularly rich in essential fatty acids, suggesting an underlying need for tissue replacement and repair. In animal experiments, diets deficient in essential fatty acids have led to the development of kidney tumours. Humans with bladder cancer have low plasma levels of arachidonic and omega-3 fatty acid metabolites. And in a placebo-controlled study on transplant patients, grafts survived better in those treated with evening primrose oil.

Gastrointestinal disorders: Earlier in this chapter the point was made that one role of essential fatty acids is to control the flow of water through certain tissues, including those of the intestine. This flow happens during normal digestion; but, during illness it may be abnormally fast or slow. Irritable bowel syndrome (IBS) is an uncomfortable condition in which fluid flow is disrupted by an unknown series of events or circumstances. Clinical treatment with essential fatty acids has been tried to relieve IBS symptoms. However, while some success has been achieved, the picture is not consistent. Gamma-linolenic acid seems to have little effect, unless bowel symptoms are associated with PMS. More hopeful are results from trials involving ulcerative colitis, where inflammation may be a more central problem. While much research remains to be done, there is good reason to believe that the next decade will see more and better treatment for bowel symptoms, using essential fatty acid derivitives.

In conclusion

Over the past decade, scientists have explored a subcellular approach to disease prevention and therapy. Many major medical advances have expanded our understanding of the molecular form and functions of cell structures in the human body, and how they relate to health and disease. Work with proteins and the DNA pattern of the genetic code generated considerable excitement. Now, however, the way ahead is certain to include essential fatty acids as well.

In today's world, fat is no longer a forbidden topic. The appropriate intake of essential fatty acids in our diet, and the development of medical products from these fats are means of achieving a long and productive life. Our individual responsibility now is to know how to select and use these powerful substances.

chapter five

THE COOK, THE KITCHEN
AND SOME BOTTLES OF OIL:
TIPS FOR HEALTHY EATING

GOOD nutrition is about good food. This makes the kitchen your first stop in changing the balance of fats you and your family eat. By adjusting your attitude towards fats and oils, and getting to know more about buying, storing and using them, you can enjoy some of the most exciting natural flavours on offer. At the same time you can be sure that you are satisfying your body's need for essential fatty acids.

You might think that my encouraging you to *increase* the amount of fat in your diet is somewhat strange in a book devoted to good health and the prevention of illness. But, consider what we have learned so far:

• We are not talking about just any fat in this book. We are focused on those universal, delicate, bendable molecules – essential fatty acids – and research shows that essential fatty acids are vital to the structure and well-being of our bodies. Many scientists believe that when illness, very-low-fat weight-loss diets, and various forms of lifestyle stress cause the level of essential fatty acids to fall below our body's requirements, degenerative diseases can result. In other words, *ESSENTIAL FATTY ACIDS ARE THE FATS WE NEED TO EAT.*

• EFAs are a natural part of many fresh food products, and the best natural sources are plant seeds and fruits, and oily fish. They are found in highest concentrations in food products linked with fast growth and new cell development.

• Because essential fatty acids are delicate, their biologically active structure can be altered by processes used in the manufacture of food products. An example is the hydrogenation process that hardens oils for margarine. The *trans*-fatty acids found in the fat content of most processed foods compete with the natural *cis*-form of polyunsaturated fatty acids, and increase our requirement for them. By learning to use products high in natural polyunsaturated fats in our foods prepared at home, we can reduce our exposure to *trans*-fats.

• And, finally, for good health and to help fight heart disease, rheumatoid arthritis, cancer, hypertension, and a number of other degenerative diseases, we need to increase the proportion of unsaturated to saturated fats we eat. Cutting down saturated fats is not enough. That is a healthy first step, but it must be followed by increasing our intake of unsaturated fats.

But, fats make you fat! If I eat too many unsaturated fats, I'll gain weight!

That's true. When eaten in excess, even essential fatty acids will cause you to gain weight. Just like their saturated cousins, unsaturated fats, including the essential fatty acids, contain approximately 9 calories of energy per gram. If your total intake of calories – from fats, carbohydrates and proteins – exceeds the amount you use as energy during the day, your body will thriftily store the remainder away as fat. While essential fatty acids are basic to good health, too much of the beautiful foods containing them can add inches to your waistline.

Watch your total calorie intake if you are watching your weight. And remember – there is nothing 'magic' in the word CALORIE. A calorie is a measure of heat energy: nothing more. Using energy burns calories. That is why exercise helps you lose those extra pounds.

Don't let anyone try to mislead you into believing there are 'good' and 'bad' calories. Because all energy from all types of food is the same, there is only one type of calorie.

Let's get back to the kitchen

Fats and oils are vital in cooking because they lend their own unique flavours to foods, and add to the pleasurable sensations of eating. To prove these points, all you need to do is eat one half of a piece of plain, dry toast, then lightly butter and taste the second half. The smooth sensation of the butter in your mouth, plus the particular taste of the unique combination of fatty acids and milk proteins in the spread makes the taste experience very different indeed. Or, try making a vegetable soup – a minestrone, perhaps – but completely avoid any ingredient containing fat or oil. The taste and texture may be very pleasing and, if the soup is made correctly, should be. However, by adding olive oil to the soup the character of its texture, aroma and flavour will all be changed for the better.

Cooking methods – such as frying, roasting and sautéeing – are all about changing food taste and food texture by applying heat in different ways. Fats and oils are important in the cooking process because of the way they help transfer heat. For example, a slice of rare beef steak fried quickly in a pan containing a small amount of oil or butter, differs greatly in taste and texture from a similar piece which has been steamed or poached. Boiled potatoes are different in taste and texture from those quickly deep-fried in an appropriate oil. By altering the type of fat used in cooking, the total appearance and quality of food can be changed.

Notice the use of the word 'appropriate'. Different oils and fats conduct and respond to heat differently because they contain different substances. The fatty acids in butter, for example, are almost all short-chain saturates. However, butter is only about 82 per cent fat. It also contains milk protein and some water, which is why it spits and burns when left too long over a high flame. When the water and milk protein are removed by a process known as 'clarification', the pure butter fat can withstand very high cooking temperatures without smoking. This is because most of its fatty acids are made up of short, saturated carbon chains. The most famous of these is butyric acid, which gives butter its 'buttery' flavour. For many dishes, including some of the best French sauces, this pure butter, made from bovine milk, is particularly important in developing their distinctive flavours. Ghee, a clarified butter fat most often made from buffaloes' milk, is used extensively in Indian cooking and helps give a distinctive flavour to that cuisine.

Refined olive oil contains almost nothing except fatty acids, a high percentage of which is oleic acid, a monounsaturate. This oil can withstand high temperatures for considerable periods of time, which makes it an excellent medium for certain types of deep frying. However, extra fine virgin oil obtained from the first, cold-pressing of the fruits – the kind of oil that is very green and has the distinctive smell and taste of olives – cannot be heated to a high temperature for long before it begins to smoke. That is the sign the products in the oil are breaking down and changing, and should send up a red flag to the cook. Which oil you choose – refined or extra virgin – depends on what you are preparing. If it is a salad, or plate of pasta dressed in oil and Parmesan cheese, reach for the extra virgin variety. If, however, you are preparing deep-fried vegetables, use the refined oil. It will withstand the high heat needed to quickly seal in and preserve the flavours of watery beets, lettuce and similar vegetables.

Asian cooks, especially Chinese, use much more oil than most of their western counterparts. Typically, a small amount of soya or peanut oil is poured into a metal pan and heated before other ingredients are added. The hot oil seals the surface of the vegetables or meats being cooked. This captures the fresh flavour of the food, and adds the special taste of the outer, slightly caramelized outer layer.

There are a few cases where overheating oil is used to achieve a unique flavour. For example, Indian cooks heat mustardseed oil until it begins to give off a slight haze. At this point, the pungent flavour of the raw oil changes to a sweet flavour we associate with many Indian dishes. But, be warned – except for the case mentioned above, and one or two others – when cooking oil smokes, it is too hot. As the changing flavour of heated mustardseed oil suggests, the chemical nature of the oil also changes.

Working in your own kitchen, you may have also noticed that different oils behave differently after they are heated. Some may thicken, and the smell and flavour may become very unpleasant.

That is because heat – especially when accompanied by the presence of extraneous carbohydrates and proteins from food such as potatoes, or fish in batter – causes alterations in the structure of fatty acids. This includes oxidation of the fats, and the development of *trans*-fats and abnormal chain structures between fat molecules. There is good reason to believe that some of these unnatural substances are responsible for the stomach upsets experienced by some people after eating fatty fried foods.

Fatty acids containing points of unsaturation in their carbon chain are most susceptible to these changes. When choosing an oil, remember that the higher the concentration of polyunsaturated fatty acids, the lower the temperature at which the oil will begin to change. Consequently, certain oils – safflower and sunflower, for example – are not good choices for deep frying. This is counter to advice in some cookery books, but just think about the logic for a minute. Instead, try corn and peanut oils – they will thicken less, can be filtered and reused more times, and will stay fresh-tasting.

There was a time when refined cottonseed oil was favoured by many cooks: it added neither flavour nor colour of its own to the food, and could be heated to a high temperature with little trouble. However, over the past few years, scientists monitoring the purity of the oil found traces of pesticides in some samples. The problem has been corrected; but such is the history of foods in our modern age.

Facts about the characteristics of popular cooking oils are presented in the table on the next page, and more detailed information is provided in appendix a: Fat Composition of Selected Foods. The latter contains lists of the types of fats present in a number of food products, including meats, prepared foods and a variety of oils, seed and nuts.

Characteristics of cooking oils

Type of oil	Characteristics	Smoke point *	Saturated fats ***	Mono-unsaturated fats**	Poly-unsaturated fats****
Almond oil	Clear, bland flavour, good for dressings	High			
Canola (Rapeseed) oil (refined)	Neutral flavour, good for frying & deep frying	High	Low	High	High
Canola oil (roasted seeds)	Distinctive meaty taste, good for sauces	? Best used at lower temperatures	? Some *trans*-fats may be present	?	?
Cottonseed	Bland taste	High	Low	Low	High
Corn oil (refined)	Excellent for all types of cooking, almost neutral taste, imparts golden colour to food	High	Low	Moderate	High
Corn oil (unrefined)	Excellent nutty flavour, golden colour	Use only at medium heat or lower	?	?	?
Grapeseed	Neutral taste, use in all types of cooking & frying	?	?	?	?
Hazelnut oil	Use at medium to low heat; excellent in sauces	Low to moderate	?	?	?
Olive oil/ extra virgin (unrefined)	Dark green colour, distinctive smell & taste, excellent in sauces, salads, pastas, etc	Low to moderate heat	?	?	?
Olive oil (refined)	Lighter colour, more neutral taste and smell	High to moderate	Low	High	Low

Characteristics of cooking oils

Type of oil	Characteristics	Smoke point *	Saturated fats ***	Mono-unsaturated fats**	Poly-unsaturated fats****
Peanut oil	Yellow colour, mild, nutty taste. Good for all types of cooking, including deep-frying	High	Low	High	Moderate
Safflower oil	Light colour, neutral taste. Gives good result in all types of cooking	Can be used at high temperatures, but limit re-use	Low	Low	High
Sesame oil (refined)	Adds distinctive mild taste	High	Low	Moderate	Moderate
Sesame oil (toasted)	Very distinctive taste often used in oriental foods. Frequently used in combination with more neutral tasting oils	Moderate to low; not a good choice for deep-frying	Low	Moderate	Low
Sunflower oil	Very light colour, neutral flavour	Moderate; best for pan-frying & sautéeing	Low	Moderate	Moderate
Walnut oil	Dark colour; distinctive taste. Excellent for adding flavour to dressings & sauces	Low temperatures	?	?	?

* Smoke point: high – above 490° F (254°C); moderate – below 400°F (204°C); low – below 250°F (121°C)

** Saturated fats: high – above 50 per cent; moderate – 20/50 per cent; low – less than 20 per cent

*** Monounsaturated fats: high – above 50 per cent; moderate – 20/50 per cent; low – less than 20 per cent

**** Polyunsaturated fats: high – above 50 per cent; moderate – 20/50 per cent; low – less than 20 per cent

More specific information is available about these products in Appendix a: Fat Composition of Selected Foods

Words into practice

Unfortunately, there is usually a yawning gap between the perfect world of food and cooking as displayed on the printed page, or from the well-ordered kitchen of a television studio, and the reality most of us experience at home. In the ideal situation, there is always enough storage space in the refrigerator and on the shelves. There are never small amounts of this or that expensive ingredient left in the bottom of a box or bottle, and the family food budget is infinite. The following are some food facts and ideas that may help you select and use fats and oils more effectively in your cooking and at the table.

Why buy expensive oils when cheaper brands seem to be less trouble?

Compared to a decade ago, cooks now have a wealth of beautiful oils to choose from. These range from the highly flavoured 'toasted' seed oils (sesame and rapeseed, for example) through the expensive and delicate unrefined nut oil, and on to the economical blends of highly refined mixed vegetable oils.

Most fresh oils have some distinctive characteristic that can make a world of difference in your cooking. For deep frying, blended and refined oils are good value. For marinating, or making salad dressings in which you do not want the taste of the oil to dominate, grapeseed oil is an excellent choice. On the other hand, by adding a few drops of fresh hazelnut oil to a pâté, or by blending a few drops of fresh hazelnut oil into biscuit dough, you add a new dimension to both the smell and taste of your final product.

What is all the fuss about olive oil?

The medicinal properties of olive oil have been extolled since ancient times, when it was used to sooth burns, promote wound healing, cure insomnia, treat ulcers, and reduce the ageing appearance of skin. Today, some people continue to believe in these benefits, although in some cases there is little evidence to support the claims. Nonetheless, a great deal of excitement has been generated by observations concerning the rate of heart disease and certain types of cancer among people living in places where a bottle of olive oil is as popular on the table as a bottle of Chianti.

Olive oil is a major food ingredient throughout the Mediterranean area, where about 80 per cent of total calories consumed come from olive oil and grain products, such as pasta and bread. Here, the population has much lower rates of a number of degenerative diseases than in the rest of Europe or the United States. In contrast to people living around the Mediterranean Sea, the average American, for instance, consumes about 70 per cent of his or her calories from saturated fats and proteins.

A hot debate is in progress about what protective effect, if any, olive oil really has. Some medical scientists believe differences in rates of heart disease and cancer are related to the amount of the monounsaturated fat (oleic acid) contained in olive oil: about 70 per cent. This school of thought is based on research linking high levels of dietary oleic acid with lowered levels of dangerous low-density blood cholesterol. In most of these studies, levels of protective high-density blood cholesterol have remained high. By contrast, experiments using polyunsaturated oils alone show these fatty acids are lower in both low- and high-density cholesterol. The facts about the biochemistry behind these changes remain obscure.

Other investigators believe that the real reason for this difference in heart disease rates rests in the ratio of saturated fatty acids to omega-6 fatty acids. Basically, the theory is that high levels of monounsaturated fats in foods reduces the level of saturated fats consumed, and thereby increases the relative amount of essential fatty acids to saturated fats.

But, while scientists sort out why the sunny shores of the Mediterranean produce so many healthy octogenarians, the Italians, Portuguese and French are lacing their food with a variety of olive oils because it tastes so good. Try it for yourself. Dip some freshly baked bread in a pool of fresh, green virgin olive oil, and see what you think.

Olive oils are as distinctive as wines. In fact, in many French shops you can buy your olive oil along with your wine, selecting both for the unique flavour and scent of the region in which their base fruits were grown. If you have not tried taste-testing olive oils, do so. You will find some oils that are peppery, while others carry a sweet smell that may remind you of summer foliage. Try pouring a little oil from Tuscany, or Provence, in the hollow of your hand between your extended thumb and forefinger. Smell its lush, almost floral aroma; then taste some. There are people who find good olive oil so enjoyable they drink it straight, like a good whisky!

But beware, olive oil has its place. On pasta, in dips, over salads and grilled fish – it is wonderful. This may not be the case in a delicate soufflé, or roulard, however.

What should I keep in mind when I buy oils for cooking?

• Buy the best quality you can afford.

• Buy in small quantities, and follow the sell-by and use-by dates. Even when given special attention, oils high in poly-unsaturated fats will oxidize over time.

• Make sure the cap or cork can be tightly secured.

• If your budget allows, buy several types, so you can enjoy the range of flavours and textures they can add to your food.

How should I store oils rich in mono- and polyunsaturated fatty acids?

Delicate oils are best kept tightly closed, in a cool, dark place to help reduce the rate of oxidation. Many oils are sold in cans to protect them from light.

In her book, *The Way to Cook*, Julia Child, the American doyenne of French cooking, claims to keep her most delicate oils – such as unprocessed fresh avocado, walnut and peanut oil – in the refrigerator because they have 'gone off in taste' when left out.

Unless you live in a warm climate, for most cooking oils a dark shelf in a cool part of the kitchen is adequate.

What do the terms 'virgin' and 'cold–pressed' mean?

Oils have been extracted from fruits and seeds for millennia by using the simple process of crushing and pressing. If you have made peanut butter at home, you will know how much oil can be released from a handful of crushed peanuts, and the same is true for sesame seed, rape seed, hazelnut, corn, olives – even avocado.

The most flavourful and distinctively coloured oil is produced by the first pressing, which is done without adding heat. This first, 'cold' pressed, 'virgin' product commands the highest price because of its unique characteristics. 'Extra virgin oil' commands an even higher price, because it contains few of the possible contaminants that may accompany the first flow of oil from the initial pressing. A special stream of oil is collected after the oil has begun to flow.

However, after that first pressing, more oil remains in the fruit or seed pulp, and it makes good commercial sense to extract as much as possible. By applying heat, and in some cases, chemicals, an additional yield is obtained. Sometimes two, three, or more extractions are possible. These produce oils which have less uniqueness in their character, and are lighter in appearance.

How can I tell if oil has oxidized?

Smell it. If it has a nasty, rather fishy tang to it – discard it. That may be heartbreaking, because good oils are expensive; but rancid oils will only damage the flavour and smell of the food you are about to prepare, and the oxidized oils are no good for your body.

How many times can I use oil for deep-frying, and how should I care for oil after use?

Experts do not agree on this topic. Some say oil should be used, filtered and reused no more than five times. Others say that this process can be repeated up to 12 times, if proper filtration methods are followed. If you ask me, I use oil only once or twice for deep frying, because fresh always tastes better.

Ultimately, the best advice is to use your own judgement.

What happens to your cooking oil when you deep fry depends on what kind of oil you are using, the maximum temperature to which it is heated, how long it is kept hot, and how it is cared for after use.

The fats in oils are altered by heat and the oxygen in the air. There is evidence that some of these changes create *trans*-fatty acids, and other branched fatty acids, which may be difficult to digest. Some scientists believe these fats add to the danger of heart disease.

You can tell when fats have been damaged by heat because there is an increased 'thickness' (viscosity) when they are poured. More telling, you may detect the sudden appearance of an unpleasant fishy odour, because some of the molecules of oil have oxidized and become rancid.

Light oils that contain high proportions of polyunsaturated fatty acids should not be used for frying at high temperature as they break-down quickly. Refined olive oil, on the other hand, can be used several times at high temperatures. Always filter oil after it has been used and cooled, and store it in a sealed container to avoid further exposure to the air.

Are cooking oils really that different?

Yes! Although they may appear much alike when they are lined up in bottles or cans on a supermarket shelf, oils offer a range of qualities that can affect your cooking.

• First, as discussed earlier, the fatty acids composition of oils differs, making them higher or lower in their level of saturated, monounsaturated and polyunsaturated fatty acids.

• Second, largely because the types of fatty acids they contain, some cooking oils withstand heat better then others. The critical factor is the temperature at which an oil begins to smoke. When that occurs, it is not a good medium in which to prepare food. Peanut oil, also known as groundnut oil, can withstand temperatures up to 200°C, or 390°F, and is therefore an excellent choice for deep frying. Proper filtration, through muslin or cheesecloth, after use makes it possible to reuse this oil several times. Sunflower oil, by contrast, begins to smoke at a much lower temperature, and should only be used for low-temperature frying, or in dressings.

• Third, most oils – particularly cold-pressed and refined, also known as virgin, oils – not only contain a mixture of fatty acids specific to their source, but also traces of other natural products found in the nuts or seeds from which they are produced. These differences provide distinct flavours that can be used to enhance our food. Experiment with different types of oils in your cooking. Try walnut oil in pastry. Or, as its flavour can be quite powerful, try a 1:1 mixture of walnut and corn oil as a dressing for green salads. Torn spinach leaves, thinly sliced white mushroom and grated hard boiled egg make an exceptional salad when tossed with a hazelnut and lime vinaigrette, to which you have added some salt, pepper, and a tiny portion of dry mustard.

Should I stop cooking with butter?

No, but keep the servings as small as possible. Part of the problem with many diets today is that they make us feel deprived. Using fats sensibly is part of creating a diet that is both healthy and delicious.

Butter has a special place in cooking. It has a wonderful affect on the tongue and mouth when we chew, and the milk proteins it contains help to stimulate our salivary gland. It gives a taste and texture to foods that cannot be matched by any substitute. Just remember – butter has that lovely, firm texture when first taken from the refrigerator because it mainly consists of short-chain, saturated fats. To cut down the amount of saturated fat in your diet, you need to use this tempting substance sparingly.

Four ways to make a little butter go a long way are:

• Make your own butter-oil spread. Buy good quality, unsalted butter and some refined grapeseed oil. Because butter is very hard when it is cold, cut off a piece weighing about 100g (approx. 4 oz) and let it come to room temperature. When it is soft, blend in an equal volume of oil. Taste and salt. If you wish, you can add flavouring at this point: lemon oil and freshly ground black pepper are good for cooking. Place the mixture in a suitable container, refrigerate and allow to stand overnight. You have cut the quantity of saturates approximately by half, added much needed polyunsaturates, and eliminated the possibility of introducing *trans*-fatty acids. Just remember, you have not reduced the number of calories.

• For spreading on toast, let the butter come to room temperature before you use it. Use a little on hot toast, and make it go a long way.

• A small amount of butter carries considerable taste. If you are sautéeing fish or meat and want that special butter taste, use a blend of two-thirds corn or peanut oil and one-third butter. Use a non-stick pan with the smallest amount of total fat possible to achieve the flavour you desire.

• For vegetables, such as green beans, melt a small portion of butter and coat the inside of the serving dish. Toss the vegetables with seasoning as soon as they are placed in the dish.

What about lard, and dripping?

Use these in careful moderation. Each type of cooking fat brings its own special characteristics to foods. Lard gives a special taste to special foods. For example, many of the best cooks argue that lard is essential for good pie-crust. See how you feel about this for yourself. Try making crust using a vegetable-oil based recipe, and then decide whether or not you think lard makes that much difference. If so, make pie-crust rarely, and remember that you have had a good size dose of saturated fat.

As for dripping, this is often used by cooks to carry a meaty flavour into a less attractive food. Unfortunately, like butter, dripping is almost pure saturated fat. Find a substitute. And, again, if you succumb, or you can't avoid eating them during Sunday lunch at your Mum's, remember to adjust your diet for the next day or two to make up the difference.

I hate cooking oily fish!

You are not alone. The smell can be unpleasant and hang about the kitchen after the fish itself is long gone. To get the omega-3 fatty acids your body needs, however, oily fish are an important part of your diet. Consider the following:

• Use food supplements containing omega-3 fatty acids. This can be expensive, and natural sources are always best.

• The fresher the fish the less oil is released from its flesh. Buy fish as close to the time you plan to serve it as possible.

• When you buy fish, do not forget to also buy lemons. Squeeze fresh lemon juice over the fish before grilling, barbecuing or frying, and save the remaining skin and fleshy parts to rub over knives, cooking utensils, and your hands to remove lingering fish oil.

• Try pickling, or marinating, fresh herring and other small, oily fish.

• Avoid cooking oily fish in batter, try grilling instead. Take a tip from the French, and brush fresh herring with a mixture of mustard and olive oil, tuck a piece of fresh parsley, rosemary or basil inside, and place over a hot outdoor grill. Turn the fish as soon at you can see the upper surface begin to pale, and cook for two or three minutes on the other side; then test with a fork to make certain it is cooked down to the bone. In other words – cook it hot, cook it fast, and cook it completely.

• Try this method for getting the most enjoyment from fresh salmon: Heat an oven to 200°C (390°F). For each serving, lightly oil a sheet of baking parchment and place two or three slices of lemon in its centre. Arrange some fresh dill over the lemon and top with a slice of fresh salmon, about one inch thick. Add a few grains of freshly ground black pepper. Pour a very small amount of olive oil in the centre of the fish and top with a slice of fresh lime. Add a few leaves of any fresh herb – parsley, thyme or basil. Bring up the sides of the parchment together and form into a package over the fish, giving it room to breath. 'Pin' shut with a toothpick. Place the parcel on a metal tray that has been heating in the oven; bake at 200°C (390°F) for 15 minutes. Serve hot with boiled potatoes and green vegetables, or allow to cool, refrigerate and serve as the centrepiece of a cold salad dressed with a very small quantity of home made mayonnaise. The combined flavours of the citrus fruit and herbs complement the taste of the salmon, making a dressing or mayonnaise almost unnecessary.

Don't forget the nuts!

Nuts and seeds are not only an excellent source of the health oils we should incorporate into our cooking, they also are rich sources of vitamin E, minerals and other substances needed for normal growth and health. Clever cooks can add both creativity and nutrient value to their food by using freshly roasted nuts and seeds to the foods they create. Table 4, in Appendix a, provides specific information about selected edible seeds and nuts. The next chapter, on antioxidants, contains specific tips on their use and health benefits.

Any last words?

Yes. According to the latest thinking on fats in our diet, the key to health is not related to the quantity of saturated fat we eat (within reason) as much as it is to the proportion of saturated to unsaturated fats. Remember that saturated fats increase our need for essential fatty acids. Reducing the total amount of saturated fat in the foods you eat, while increasing the quantity of high-quality oils you use in food preparation, makes sense.

Finally, unrefined plant oils are used by nature to 'power up' new growing things. Take advantage of their goodness whenever you can. Buy in small quantities, and use the freshest and best you can afford.

chapter six
ANTIOXIDANTS

THIS is a book about fats. So, why include a chapter on antioxidants? The answer is simple. Antioxidants protect essential
fatty acids from the devastating effect of scavenger molecules,
called free radicals. Practically all components in the body can be
damaged by free radicals, including DNA and proteins.
However, the delicate double bonds in unsaturated fats are
especially vulnerable. Because lipids containing essential fatty
acids are so universal in tissues, and because they perform such
fundamental biological functions, damage to them has wide-
spread consequences which have been linked to a range of
degenerative illnesses.

The polyunsaturates you eat need antioxidant protection. In
fact, that is nature's way of doing things. As a general rule, high
concentrations of polyunsaturated fats in natural plant products
are accompanied by high levels of vitamin E. Safflower and sunflower oils, for example, contain more than 40mg of vitamin E
per 100g of oil. Wheatgerm oil – the very essence of new life
for the wheat plant – contains more than 130mg of this super
radical-fighter per 100g of oil. The important lesson to be
learned from this is that when you increase the level of polyunsaturated fatty acids in your diet, make certain you also
provide adequate supplies of vitamin E to protect it.

But, vitamin E is a fat-soluble vitamin, and only works in fatty
environments – such as cell membranes. What about protecting
essential fatty acids when they are in water soluble environments;
when they are attached to proteins, for example? In these cases,
vitamin C plays the role of policeman. To fully protect the
essential fatty acids in your body, you need adequate supplies of
two powerful antioxidants – vitamin E and vitamin C.

How do antioxidants protect essential fatty acids from free radical damage?

To understand the relationship between essential fatty acids and antioxidants, it is necessary to review the structure of a typical molecule. Each molecule contains a group of atoms held together by electrical charges – also called 'covalent' forces. Atoms in a molecule can be from the same element; or, more commonly, they represent different elements. How the atoms are arranged within the structure of the molecule determines its specific characteristics. Any change in the arrangement, or mix, of atoms completely changes the characteristics of the molecule.

Under normal circumstances, molecules are in electrical balance; that is, overall they carry neither a positive nor negative charge. They are 'stable'. During various biological activities, however, changes occur in the electrical balance of individual atoms within molecules. Great chunks of a molecule can remain stable, while a little side bit suddenly loses an electron and, perhaps, gets itself involved in the release of energy from another molecule; or links up with another molecule so they can both be whisked from one place to another in the bloodstream. These very active bits of molecule are known as 'radicals', and they are a normal part of life processes. Problems arise when too many of these radicals are produced – through exposure to X-rays perhaps – or because of cigarette smoke. It is these extra 'free radicals' that become nasty.

But, what is a '*free* radical'? In addition to the protons and neutrons which combine to make up the central core of atoms in a molecule, each also has a full complement of small, negatively charged, sub-atomic particles, called electrons. Electrons exist in pairs, and sometimes – in the process of a chemical interaction – an electron goes missing. At once, a molecule lacking an electron seeks to satisfy its need for covalent balance. Imbalance is unnatural and destructive.

Metaphorically, electrons are 'fickle', tending to spin off their own nicely-balanced molecule if a passing molecule attracts them to satisfy its own electron complement. A free radical can split an electron off a neighbouring molecule, making it into another hungry radical seeking an extra electron, and so on. The process of giving and taking electrons initiates a chain reaction capable of creating considerable damage in its local environment.

Nonetheless, free radical formation is an important part of normal cellular metabolism, particularly respiration. Oxygen is necessary for life to continue, and during the respiration process it is combined with hydrogen and converted to water (H_2O). However, for a variety of reasons, sometimes only one hydrogen atom attaches to the oxygen atom, and the result is an electron-hungry, superoxide radical – also known as 'reactive oxygen'. This molecule can cause significant damage.

So, why don't we dissolve into a mass of free radicals?

To guard against free radical damage, the body has a built-in safety system consisting of specific enzymes and nutrients. Molecules in all of these substances can give up an electron without becoming chemically unstable. Part of this safety system – the nutrients – includes vitamins C and E, and beta-carotene. In the case of fatty acids, vitamins C and E are the most important. The remainder of the system involves a series of protein molecules known as enzymes.

To work, enzymes need atoms of trace minerals – the most important of these are selenium, copper, iron, zinc and manganese. That is why trace minerals are necessary nutrients in the foods you eat. That is also why certain food supplements combine trace minerals with vitamins. The combined effect is better than any single ingredient of these products. Perhaps, for example, you are one of the millions of people who have found that a combination of selenium and vitamins C, E and A has helped control the symptoms of rheumatoid arthritis.

What external conditions stimulate free radical formation?

The level of free radicals in the body can be boosted by a number of circumstances – smoking cigarettes, inhaling exhaust fumes, exposure to ultra-violet radiation (too much time in the sun), excessive alcohol, certain illnesses and certain drugs.

Does that list sound familiar? It is the same as the list of conditions that block the enzyme delta-6-desaturase in the transformation of the omega-6 fatty acid, linoleic acid, to the all important gamma-linolenic acid, and the transformation of the essential omega-3 fatty acid, alpha-linolenic acid to metabolites leading up to the creation of eicosapentaenoic acid.

How are omega-6 and omega-3 fatty acids affected by free radicals?

The double bonds that give specific biological importance to the omega-6 and omega-3 series of molecules are highly susceptible to attack from free radicals. Antioxidants, such as vitamins E and C deactivate free radicals and prolong the effectiveness of the fatty acids and substances containing them.

What is vitamin E?

Vitamin E, also called alpha-tocopherol, is an oily substance found in seeds, nuts, grains and vegetable oils. Like other antioxidants, it can absorb free radicals without becoming highly reactive. It is rejuvenated quickly in the presence of adequate levels of vitamin C, and of the trace mineral, selenium.

Vitamin E protects essential fatty acids while they are in a lipid, or fatty, environment. We have much to learn about the role of vitamin E in human health. Until recently, no nutritional use to humans could be identified for this vitamin, and many people argued that the substance was basically without value in human metabolism. Now, however, medical research is demonstrating vitamin E's importance to the normal transport of cholesterol and other lipids in the blood. As these processes all involve essential fatty acids, which are highly sensitive to attack by free radicals, vitamin E has a major role in maintaining normal biological activity.

What is the link between vitamin C and essential fatty acids?

Vitamin C helps protect essential fatty acids against destruction by free radicals in watery environments. By sharing electrons, vitamin C regenerates vitamin E, enabling it to continue protecting essential fatty acids in cell membranes and other fatty substances.

Vitamin C enhances a number of chemical reactions involving lipid molecules that stimulate the synthesis of prostaglandin PGE1, which is anti-inflammatory, and inhibit the production of prostaglandin PGE2, a substance known to increase inflammation.

Does vitamin C fight cancer and other degenerative diseases? If so, how?

Nobel laureate, Linus Pauling spent most of his later years fighting to convince conventional medical science of the medical importance of vitamin C. At first his championing of vitamin C was scorned, and by the late 1980s his work in nutrition was thought by many to be completely discredited. About that time, however, a separate group of investigators began publishing evidence from large population studies suggesting that several natural antioxidants, including vitamins C and E, have a significant inverse correlation with the rate of certain types of cancer and coronary heart disease. In other words, people consuming higher levels of these natural antioxidants have less chance of developing cancer and heart disease.

Many scientists now believe that vitamin C scavenges free radicals and protects unsaturated fats against peroxidation, thereby reducing the cellular damage that can lead to abnormal cell growth and cancer.

Is there a link between antioxidants and the ageing process?

It is well known that essential fatty acids, DNA (deoxyribonucleic acid) and RNA (ribonucleic acid) molecules are all highly susceptible to damage by an accumulation of free radicals. It is thought that these cause alterations in the composition and structure of cell membranes, the structure of genetic material controlling cell division, the passage of material across cell membranes, and certain specific steps in metabolism. Overall, when bombarded by large amounts of free radicals over time, cells are disabled and die or fail to properly perform their metabolic functions.

A growing body of research suggests antioxidants slow this process. Ageing is a major cause of cataracts, or clouding of the eye lens. Several large international studies have demonstrated significant reduction in common age-related cataracts when antioxidants were taken as part of a daily routine over time.

The cosmetics industry has capitalized on the beneficial effects of vitamin E, and included this antioxidant in skin and body products to help slow the signs of ageing.

How can I increase the amounts of natural vitamin C in my diet?

Refer to Appendix b in this book to identify foods rich in this important antioxidant. Then look through your cookery books to find new ways to enjoy including these foods in your normal diet. But remember, vitamin C is fragile, and cooking heat destroys it. Look for ways to use these ingredients raw wherever possible. Be inventive. For example:

Make refreshing drinks with fresh lemons, oranges or limes. Home-made lemonade and iced tea flavoured with orange juice boost your daily intake of vitamin C.

Serve exotic fruit salads for dessert – try guava and melon, or combine strawberries and mango. Another pleasant end to a meal is a light, refreshing lime or fresh kiwi sorbet.

Half-a-cup of chopped green pepper contains almost 100mg of vitamin C. Use ultra thin strips of the vitamin-packed vegetable to add colour and crunch to salads.

Batons of red and green peppers kept chilled in a container of water in the refrigerator make good 'pick-me-up' snacks. Add some strips of young carrots for variety in taste and colour.

Try using more freshly-squeezed lemon and lime juice in salad dressings, and in cold dressings for fish and cold cooked poultry dishes.

Enjoy fresh strawberries sliced and served with a sprinkle of brown sugar in a crystal glass, or on top of thin crêpes dusted with sweet cocoa powder.

Enjoy blackcurrants by including them as an edible garnish on your plate, as the key ingredient in home-made sorbets, and as part of that good English tradition – Summer Pudding.

What evidence is there that vitamin E may reduce heart disease?

A considerable number of scientific papers exist on this subject, but some of the most convincing evidence comes from two studies published in the May 1993 issue of the *New England Journal of Medicine*. Medical investigators in the United States monitored about 40,000 men and 80,000 women over periods of four and eight years, respectively. Both men and women taking daily vitamin supplements containing at least 100 international units of vitamin E per day showed significant reduction in risk from heart diseases. However, this research demonstrated little protective benefit from dietary sources, thus suggesting the importance of food supplements.

How can I increase the amount of vitamin E in my diet?

Research nutritionists experimenting with antioxidants suggest we should consume between 50 and 80mg of vitamin E each day. Others recommend much higher levels if your diet is rich in polyunsaturated oils, or if your environment makes you highly susceptible to free radical exposure.

Many foods are rich in vitamin E, but the amounts they contain are relatively small, therefore making it necessary to consume rather large quantities. Broccoli, spinach and Brussels sprouts will increase your dietary level of this important fat-soluble vitamin without adding too many calories. Several servings of these vegetables each day will undoubtedly be of benefit.

However, the best natural sources of vitamin E are calorie-rich nuts, seeds and oily fruits. For example, on average 100g (4 oz) of Brussels sprouts will provide 1mg of vitamin E; 25g (1 oz) of sunflower seeds will provide 10mg. A tablespoonful of wheatgerm oil contains 18mg; 30g (just over 1 oz) of almonds provide

7mg. To increase the quantities of vitamin E-rich foods in your diet, try the following:

• Use fresh sunflower and safflower seed oils in salad dressings.

• Lightly oven toast sunflower or sesame seeds and use them for crunch in salads, add them to meatloaf and burgers; try them as toppings on ice cream, fruit crumbles and yogurt desserts.

What is beta-carotene?

Beta-carotene is one of a group of natural plant pigments that give many vegetables and fruits their yellow, orange or red hue. In fact, it got its name because of the colour it imparts to carrots. Carotenes also occur in green plants, but their presence is masked by the colour of chlorophyll. If you have had the pleasure of visiting the north-eastern seaboard of the United States and Canada in autumn, you probably have observed the blaze of red and golden hues that appear as leaves die and their chlorophyll disappears.

More than 40 carotenoids occur in nature, and all are precursors of vitamin A. However, beta-carotene is the most abundant and is most actively transformed into the vitamin. Because of this, it is called *provitamin A*.

Until relatively recently, beta-carotene's capacity as a provitamin was thought to be its main benefit. However, research has shown that it has other health values. Large epidemiological studies suggest that beta-carotene lowers the risk of certain cancers. Other research, based on the use of dietary supplements, suggests a possible protective role also against heart disease.

What about beta-carotene and the immune system?

The immune system has two roles – to kill invading microbes, and to kill tumour cells. A number of experiments in animals and humans have shown that beta-carotene stimulates both of these immune responses. This suggests a role for beta-carotene in fighting infection and cancer.

How can I increase the amount of natural beta-carotene in my diet?

Recent medical research suggests we need between 6 and 15mg of beta-carotene per day. Check the list of carotene-rich foods listed in Appendix b to see which you already enjoy on a regular basis, and which you may want to include more often. If some of the items listed are new to you, experiment. Try a new taste!

Make buying carotene-rich food a part of your routine meal planning. When shopping for food, think about long, hot summer days. Buy red, orange and deep-green fruits and vegetables such as mangoes, carrots, red peppers, tomatoes, apricots, sweet potato and spinach. Try some of the following ways to appreciate the taste and texture of these fruits and vegetables:

• Enjoy the special crunch and sweetness of broccoli, carrots and red pepper served raw, as crudities or in salads. For example, try a cheerful salad made with sliced tomatoes, baby spinach leaves, and slivers of red pepper: dress with lemon juice and safflower oil, and top with a sprinkling of toasted sunflower seeds. Add a slice of cold salmon, or a piece of chicken breast, and you have a perfect summer meal.

• Learn to love carrots. In France, the culinary centre of the world, finely shredded carrots, known as *carottes râpé*, is found in almost all supermarkets. When mixed alone with a simple vinaigrette, or combined with raisin and toasted nuts, grated carrots become a delicious and interesting addition to both luncheon and dinner menus.

• Go for colourful desserts: mango sorbet, apricot and low-fat yogurt purée, for example. Pies made with sweet potato or pumpkin also boost your carotene intake, but have more calories.

Is beta-carotene safe?

According to experts, no toxicity has been demonstrated for beta-carotene, even at high levels taken over a long period of time. Beta-carotene which is not converted into vitamin A may be deposited in body fat, particularly that layer just below the skin and, if taken in very large quantities, may cause a yellowing of the skin. This can be quickly differentiated from yellowing caused by jaundice, which also colours the eyes. Also, coloration caused by beta-carotene disappears when the compound is no longer consumed.

What about selenium?

Selenium in one of the metal elements which, in very small quantities, acts as a catalyst in many important metabolic processes. For example, it helps vitamin E neutralize the free radicals that attack and deactivate essential fatty acids.

Selenium found in plants comes from the soil in which they are grown. However, soil composition varies from location to location, and there are natural deficiencies in some areas. People living in these locations should consider supplementing their daily diet with one of several commercial products combining selenium with vitamins B, C and A. (In many vitamin products, vitamin A is included instead of beta-carotene.)

Can I consume too many antioxidants?

I am not aware of any scientific study demonstrating a risk from antioxidants as a group. However, it is possible to consume too much vitamin A. Because it is a fat-soluble substance, excessive vitamin A accumulates in body tissues and can cause a condition called hypervitaminosis A. This condition is characterized by headache, hair loss, menstrual disturbances and, in extreme cases, damage to the liver and spleen. Beta-carotene, the pro-vitamin form of vitamin A, is a more effective antioxidant than the vitamin itself, and appears to be less toxic in large quantities because it is water soluble, and any excess is shed in the urine, making beta-carotene a good choice for food supplements.

There is no evidence that vitamin E is toxic in humans; and the work of Linus Pauling on vitamin C, as well as subsequent research, indicates levels as high as 3 to 5g of Vitamin C per day are safe.

Again, a word of warning: Very large doses of selenium can be toxic.

Can diet alone provide adequate quantities of antioxidants?

Yes, under certain conditions. If you consistently enjoy a blend of the fresh vegetables, fruits, fish and oils diet which experts now call the Mediterranean diet, and have no special physical illness, or suffer from unusual stress, a well-balanced diet is an enjoyable way to meet your body's needs for antioxidants. Such a diet should be high in olive oil, fish, green vegetables and foods rich in vitamin C, and it should contain limited quantities of saturated fats and small amounts of refined sugars and processed foods.

However, if you smoke, are unwell, use certain medications, or are under considerable physical and mental stress, then taking an antioxidant food supplement each day may be of considerable benefit in reducing your risk of developing a chronic disease.

chapter seven

THE DIET DILEMMA

DIETING is big business. If you look in the mirror and think your skirt is getting a bit tight at the hip, you can rest assured there are thousands of people producing tapes, giving television interviews, selling boxes and cans of diet products, and yes – even writing books – to help you put things right. It is all a little mad. In the affluent western world we live in, although some people starve through poverty, most of us worry about gaining weight. Social pressures, fashion trends – even health warnings encourage people to put down their forks and take off the pounds.

But food is pleasurable; food is beautiful. Sharing food is an important means of communication. Social reasons make it difficult to cut down what we eat. Even more important, dieting is a bore! And, to make matters worse, medical experts say some diets provide inadequate quantities of certain nutrients, and that some others can be harmful. That results in a diet dilemma. If we want to change our eating habits for health reasons, or to loose weight and meet some personal goal, how can we tell which diets are palatable, effective – and nutritionally sound?

Good diets/bad diets – what is the difference?

A good diet is a balanced diet. It contains good sources of protein, a high proportion of unrefined starches – such as pasta and wholemeal bread – and *it includes* fat. Wherever possible, it incorporates fresh foods, freshly prepared.

In 1994, the international journal *Nutrition Reviews* published the following table comparing dietary guidelines recommended by the United States government in 1980, 1985 and 1990.

A comparison of the dietary guideline 1980, 1985, 1990

1980	1985	1990
Eat a variety of foods. Maintain ideal weight	Eat a variety of foods. Maintain desirable weight	Eat a variety of foods. Maintain healthy weight
Avoid too much fat, saturated fat and cholesterol	Avoid too much fat, saturated fat and cholesterol	Choose a diet low in fat, saturated fat and cholesterol
Eat foods with adequate starch and fibre	Eat foods with adequate starch and fibre, fruits and grain products	Choose a diet with plenty of vegetables.
Avoid too much sugar	Avoid too much sugar	Use sugar only in moderation
Avoid too much sodium	Avoid too much sodium	Use salt and sodium only in moderation
If you drink alcohol, do so in moderation	If you drink alcoholic beverages, do so in moderation	If you drink alcoholic beverages, do so in moderation

Reprinted with permission from *Nutrition Reviews* 52; 11:395.

In other words, during a decade when the diet gurus and exercise experts were selling a range of faddish eating practises, the advice from nutritionists remained the same. Moderation is the key.

It is interesting how little the actual language of the advice was modified between 1980 and 1990. Instead of becoming more rigid, as one might expect during a time of particular interest in the link between obesity and heart disease, the tone of the message actually softened. Instead of demanding 'Eat', as was the case in 1980, by 1990 the words suggested we 'Choose'. The need for individual action was clearly being respected. Nonetheless, the nutritionists' central message remained the same: eat a limited amount of fats – particularly saturated fats –

and enjoy a mix of foods containing modest amounts of sugar and salt. Any eating plan that includes these basic principles is a good one.

What about fat? How much should I eat?

First, a warning. Never put a child under the age of 5 on a low-fat diet. They need the energy. At this age, low-fat diets may restrict growth.

Fat is a necessary part of any good diet. Healthy adults need at least 30g (just over 1 oz) of fat each day to help absorb fat-soluble vitamins A, D and E, and for energy. They also need to consume oil from nuts and seeds to obtain the essential fatty acids their bodies require. Normal western diets contain 80g (3 oz) or more of fat per day, too much of which is in the form of *trans*-polyunsaturated fatty acids. It would be healthier to reduce the total fat in the diet by cutting out sources of *trans*-fats (processed foods) and focusing on good sources of polyunsaturated fats to meet the requirement for essential fatty acids.

Nutritionists believe we need at least 5g (⅕ oz) of essential fatty acid a day. This amount does not account for additional demands caused by smoking, illness, X-rays, air pollution, and so on. It also does not account for the possibility that some polyunsaturated fats we eat have been changed from *cis*- to *trans*- fatty acids during food processing or preparation. Remember, *1g of polyunsaturated oil contains less that 1g of essential fatty acid.*

Thinking about fats, what should I look for in a diet?

A good diet offers eating tips that help you cut out as much saturated fat as possible. If you enjoy red meats (which are rich in saturated fat) eat them in small amounts every now and then: NOT EVERY DAY. Be sensible. If you cannot live without salami, or an occasional piece of bacon, keep it at that – occasional. Even then, drain off as much fat as possible on to paper towelling before you put the meat on your plate.

Are all animal fats the same?

No. Fatty tissues from beef and lamb contain the highest quantities of saturated fats, while poultry and pork contain less. Diets incorporating 'white meats' contain less saturated fat than diets containing 'red meat'. The tables presented in Appendix A give examples of how the fat content of meats and other foods varies.

Do I need to eat cholesterol?

Yes. Your diet should include about a gram of cholesterol a day, which can be obtained from egg yolks and an occasional serving of meat. Cholesterol is important for the construction of cell membranes and steroid hormones, and for the formation of bile salts, which are necessary for the digestion of fats. Cholesterol also plays a key role in transporting fats from the bloodstream to the body's cells. In other words – a balanced diet should contain a little cholesterol.

Do not confuse a *low-cholesterol diet* with a *cholesterol-lowering diet*. Most cholesterol is made by cells in the liver from saturated fats. Eliminating foods containing cholesterol from your diet will have little effect on your blood cholesterol level: but switching from saturated to mono- and polyunsaturated fats will.

What about foods labelled 'low-fat' and 'no-fat'?

Such labels are useless because the terms have never been legally defined. Often the labels are little more than a marketing ploy, and the products can be expensive for the food value they contain – and some may be another source of *trans*-fatty acids. They also fulfil your need for food, thus discouraging you from enjoying the fresh, nutrient-rich foods your body should have.

If I remove all the fat from my diet, I'll lose weight. Right?

Wrong! Cutting all the fat from your diet will not keep you from gaining body fat. If you eat foods containing more energy units (calories) than you burn, your body will store that extra energy in your fat cells. That holds true for calories from bread, carrots, eggwhite, steamed white fish and anything else that goes past your lips.

How can I tell if my diet contains enough omega-6 fatty acids?

Include some fresh nuts, seeds and polyunsaturated oils in your diet each day. Linoleic acid, the key substance in the omega-6 chain of essential fatty acids occurs in fairly high quantities in walnuts and other nuts, safflower oil, soyabean oil, and linseed oil. Gamma-linolenic acid is found in oil from the seeds of a number of plants, including the evening primrose, borage (starflower) and blackcurrant. In Chapter 8 I make some suggestions about daily requirements.

Diets that specifically tell you to avoid foods rich in omega-6 and omega-3 fatty acids do not make good nutritional sense.

Should my diet contain fish?

Yes. Fish is high in protein, and oily fish – for example, herring and mackerel – contain two important omega-3 metabolites: eicosapentanoeic acid (EPA) and docosahexaenoic acid (DHA). Both have been shown to be important in reducing the risk of heart attack.

But I don't like fish – what other foods can I eat that contain omega-3 fatty acids?

Alpha-linolenic acid is the primary substance in the chain of omega-3 essential fatty acids. Good plant sources include linseed (flaxseed), pumpkin seeds, walnuts and walnut oil.

Are there other tips about diets I should avoid?

Watch out for:

• Diets containing less than 1000 calories per day for adult women and 1200 for adult men. Some experts believe this is too low for most people. If you *are* considering a diet of this

type, make certain it contains oils – on salads, for example –
and that you do not stay on it for more than a short time.

- Diets based on one food (mono-diets): bananas or pineapples
  for more than a day, for example.
- Formula diets. Look on the package. Most do not even
  mention essential fatty acids. They are expensive and are
  unlikely to provide balanced nutrition.
- Diets that exclude all, or almost all, fats. When you read over
  the diet, make certain it contains at least some oil and oily
  foods each day. Diets that cut out all seeds and nuts, and tell
  you to use oil-free salad dressing make no sense.
- Diets based on plant foods (i.e. lots of salads) but contain no
  pulses, beans, corn, wheat or rice. They are probably low in
  both proteins and essential fatty acids.
- Any diet that tells you to eat a specific food or substance
  because it will selectively 'burn fat'. You are being conned.

Are there any good diets?

Yes. Weight Watchers is one. If you use their newer generations
of recipes, and do not depend on their food products, you can
eat a well-balanced diet without spending more than your usual
food budget. There are others, but this plan represents an international resource for people who have an honest need to lose
weight.

Are there any special groups of people who should be particularly careful about fat in their diet?

Yes.

- Infants and young children need fat in their diet and should
  never be placed on a weight-reducing or low-fat diet.
- Pregnant women should make certain they consume foods
  rich in essential fatty acids.
- People with heart conditions should cut out as much saturated
  fat and *trans*-fat as possible from their diet, and increase their
  intake of oils, seeds, nuts and fish rich in essential fatty acids.

What else should I consider when I am thinking about a diet?

Consider the amount of fat-soluble antioxidants in the diet. By that, I mean vitamin E. If you increase the amount of oil and oily foods in your diet, protect them with extra vitamin E.

With so many recipe and diet books on the market, is there anything left to be said about food?

The answer is a very definite 'yes'. Relative deficiency, also called marginal malnutrition, tops the list of new food subjects that deserve attention. Various forms of this condition occur when people eat adequate quantities of food to maintain life, but not enough of one or more specific nutrients to enable them to thrive. This can happen if vegans do not carefully balance the sources of vegetable protein they eat, for example. Or, when the sick and elderly no longer feel they can eat certain types of foods. It can happen in people suffering from anorexia, and in people who diet often and to the extreme. In the early part of this book I described the links between consistently low levels of essential fatty acids in the diet and degenerative illnesses, particularly heart disease. All of these areas of nutrition are new and hold great hope for the future of many people.

Relative deficiency also occurs when people live under near-starvation conditions. Children in Africa and other parts of the world suffer from dangerously low iodine, protein and vitamin levels. Without remedy, these problems will leave us all poorer for loss of human potential.

Genetic engineering, along with modern farming methods, food processing techniques and international food transport systems are beginning to have a profound influence on what we choose to eat. This important area of food and nutrition deserves much greater public attention. We all need to understand how laws and regulations influence prices and availability of the foods we eat. The *trans*-fats debate is an example of why everyone needs to understand and know what changes food processing makes in the foods we eat each day. We need clear, understandable information – not bureaucratic gobbledegook – about the contents of the milk, the cheese, the bread, the cans of beans, and every ounce of fizzy drink and flavoured water we consume. We have the right to make informed choices. We need to have a voice in what is made available for us to eat. To have a voice, we need information.

Will there ever be a time when there are no 'diets' published in books and magazines?

That scenario is unlikely. Much has been written about how social pressures, the fashion industry and overly-zealous health claims by various 'experts' encourage people to buy and try a new diet plan at the drop of a leotard. Now, in response to years of gimmicky diets with attention-grabbing names, a new type of book has appeared. The anti-diet books *You Don't Have to Diet* by Dr Tom Sanders and Peter Bazalegette, and *Stop the Insanity* by Susan Powter are good examples. I mean GOOD, because both make good sense. Both books share a concern about misleading claims made by many diet 'experts', and they worry that too much dieting can harm even a healthy person.

As I said, these books make excellent sense. But I personally do not believe, try as they might, that the anti-diet books will ever kill off our interest in reading and trying other people's ideas about food and our bodies. The fact is that readers – particularly women – enjoy reading about diets and fashion. It is fun. It is also a way of sharing some very important parts of their lives. I believe we get involved with diets and exercise fads because they fill an important social need in our lives. If they are well presented and, perhaps, become a topic of conversation on morning television or at the hairdressers, we can participate in something important by trying them out.

There is something much more personal about reading a well-researched article describing a new diet than there is in reading an article simply explaining how to fix a roast for Sunday dinner, or how to make oatmeal biscuits. When you read a well-written diet article, it makes you feel that someone out there knows *you*; your problems; how you feel about the shape and size of your body. They marry up that understanding of you and your lifestyle with ideas concerning things you do every day – clean carrots and prepare a chicken; make a salad and sort out a fruit dessert the family enjoys. Look at it this way: someone out there *cares* about who we are and what we do.

That leaves us with the problem of credibility. We must judge what does and does not make good sense in the diet and food articles we read. While journalists and editors have the responsibility for giving us correct information, it is also up to each of us to judge whether or not a diet, or eating plan, sounds over-the-top. If it does, let the editor know. Help make sure the public will not be conned.

If you look in almost any dictionary you will see several definitions of the word 'diet'. All involve selecting and limiting foods. One diet differs from another only in the foods recommended and the proportions in which they are prepared. Take a careful look at the next diet you read, and see if it makes good sense.

chapter eight

FOOD SUPPLEMENTS

Food supplements have a fundamental place in modern nutrition. Ideally, a balanced diet containing adequate amounts of a wide range of foods, provides the nutrients you need for good health. But extra nutritional demands created by the stress and strain of today's lifestyle, and the destructive effects of food manufacturing processes, frequently make the ideal impossible.

Some time ago I watched a young woman in a health food store walk slowly up and down between two long counters of neatly arranged packages containing mineral and vitamin products. From time to time she would stop, pick up a box or bottle, read its label, put it back on the shelf and move on. After a few minutes, curiosity overcame me and I asked her what she was looking for. She shook her head in dismay and said, 'I don't know. I know I need something, but I have no idea what it is.'

Her plight reflected that of far too many people. Choosing supplements can be a difficult and costly process, and there are few places to turn for help. The woman in the health food store needed simple answers to some basic questions. Without that assistance, she would possibly waste both her time and money.

Your body's need for specific nutrients changes with age, your health status and alterations in the pattern of your daily routine. Even the composition of your diet has an effect – large amounts of saturated fats and cholesterol will increase your need for essential fatty acids, for example.

Other circumstances influencing you nutrient requirements include unusual emotional or physical stress, dieting, pregnancy, a sudden increase in your daily physical activity, injury, infection by certain viruses, a therapeutic course of prescribed drugs, certain illnesses, and lifestyle. For example, smoking, alcohol consumption, environmental pollution and excessive exposure to ultra-violet radiation, like that encountered during long bouts of sunbathing, have all been shown to increase the rate of free radical formation in otherwise healthy tissue. Free radicals damage important molecules and disrupt normal life processes. In turn, these disturbances create havoc within the body, and can lead ultimately to degenerative illnesses.

One way to increase the amount of essential nutrients, such as vitamins C and E (which help prevent the formation of excessive numbers of free radicals) is by adding foods to your diet which are known to be rich in these substances. In the case of these specific vitamins, citrus fruit and wheatgerm oil would be two good choices.

But such changes may be difficult, as the total volume of food required may be impractical; or social pressures – other family members' food preferences for example – can work against significant diet changes. Food supplements are a useful means of filling the gap. If that choice makes sense in your life, the question then is: which supplement should you choose, how much should you take, and for how long?

• A general picture •

What are food supplements?

Food supplements are commercial preparations rich in specific, natural micronutrients which have been shown to play special roles in the body's life processes. They are not pharmaceuticals, but can have a powerful influence on your general health status. Some products contain only one substance, while others contain a combination of minerals, vitamins, and complex biological compounds.

How do food supplements differ from herbal remedies?

Diet supplements should not be confused with herbal medicines. Herbal products are natural plant compounds which are not a required part of any known human biological activity. But – like pharmaceuticals – herbal products can alter these activities. The plants used to produce these products also contain vitamins and other substances found in food supplements, but their primary attraction is the presence of distinctive substances, such as volatile oils, alkaloids and flavonoids, which have known therapeutic value.

Aspirin is a good example of a widely used medication first derived from plants. Its use probably goes back as far as the classical Greek period, when extracts from a number of plants, including willow (what was to become known as aspirin was first derived from the bark of the white willow), were used for pain and fever control. Centuries later, the active plant ingredient, acetylsalicylic acid, was extracted from meadowsweet – the old botanical name for which was *Spiraea ulmaria* (hence aspirin) – which was known to contain these same medicinal properties. Advances in chemistry made it possible to duplicate the acetylsalicylic acid molecule, and the synthetic drug we now use was produced in mass quantities. Although aspirin is no longer considered to be a 'herbal' medicine, for centuries its healing relief could only be obtained from plants.

Why are food supplements necessary?

There are occasions when supplements may help. For example, when our choice of foods does not fully satisfy our body's need for specific nutrients. Also, at other times, the wear and tear of daily activities, poor appetite, slimming diets, exposure to cigarette smoke and environmental pollutants, the use of certain medications, and illness increase our need for specific nutrients. Smoking, for instance, destroys vitamin C in body tissues, and some experts believe smokers require two to three times more of this vitamin than non-smokers.

When should I take food supplements?

The first step in finding the right mix of foods and food supplements is to be able to 'listen to your body'. All of us know when we experience discomfort and pain, and most of us know when something is not quite right about the way we feel, or how well we are responding to external situations. By becoming 'tuned in' to our bodies enough to know what triggers problems, we can learn what action to take to counter the problem and relieve its symptoms.

Remember that food supplements are derived from foods and should be treated like foods. Always follow the manufacturer's instructions; but in general, food supplements should be taken with a meal. This is unlike many prescribed pharmaceuticals, which need to be taken on an empty stomach.

Is it possible to take too much?

Yes. Unfortunately some natural substances can cause trouble if taken to excess. Vitamin A is an example, which I cited earlier in the book, and prolonged use of large quantities may result in the development of a condition known as hypervitaminosis A, characterized by headache, hair loss, and irregular menstruation. In extreme cases, damage to the liver and spleen may occur.

Always follow instructions on the packaging, and always use products from reputable sources.

• Supplements containing essential fatty acids •

Why are there so many different products containing essential fatty acids?

This is a difficult question with a two-part answer.

First, products vary according to the type of unsaturated fatty acids they contain. Some contain a blend of oils high in omega-3 fatty acids, others supply large quantities of omega-6 fatty acids, and still other products contain a blend of omega-3 and omega-6 fatty acids.

Second, some products are formulated and packaged to meet a particular need. For example, some evening primrose oil products are packaged with the complex of minerals and vitamins which, through clinical investigation, have been shown to control premenstrual syndrome (PMS) in the majority of sufferers.

Does it matter if I take omega-3 or omega-6 fatty acids?

Yes. Omega-3 fatty acids, found in fish oils, have received considerable attention from the media because of scientific evidence linking diets high in these oils with low rates of heart disease. For this reason, people with a family history of heart disease, or with other reasons for concern, may choose to supplement their diet with these products.

However, extensive research has shown that omega-6 fatty acids, which are found in many plant and seed oils, have far reaching importance for all tissues in the human body. They have been shown to delay, prevent or have a positive effect on many degenerative diseases linked with the lifestyle of the western world.

When might I need to take supplements containing omega-6 fatty acids?

If you have any of the conditions I mentioned in Chapter 3, you may wish to consider trying food supplements rich in omega-6 fatty acids. These conditions include PMS, ME, arthritis, and eczema. Many people have also found that supplements containing essential fatty acids have improved the quality and appearance of their skin, hair and nails.

Will food supplements containing omega-6 fatty acids protect me against degenerative diseases?

Used in conjunction with a healthy lifestyle, proper use of food supplements containing omega-6 fatty acids will help you fight certain degenerative diseases common in western society. The connection between essential fatty acids and good health is not surprising, because omega-6-essential fatty acids are vital in the construction of the body's cells and in maintaining the local communication systems, or hormones, which link them. Scientific evidence indicates that modern lifestyles and dietary habits may increase the amount of certain forms of essential fatty acids needed for good health. Research has shown an association between reduced tissue levels of omega-6 essential fatty acids and the development of numerous non-infectious illnesses, including heart disease, PMS, mastalgia, certain skin conditions, rheumatoid arthritis, inflammation, gastric illnesses, post-viral fatigue syndrome (or ME), certain illnesses of the brain and nervous system, kidney disease and osteoporosis.

How do I know that food supplements containing omega-6 essential fatty acids are safe?

There is no scientific evidence that large amounts of natural and fresh omega-6 essential fatty acids can do harm. These substances and their metabolites – including gamma-linolenic acid and its derivatives – are normal intermediates in human metabolism, and are widely consumed in foods such as oats and human milk.

There are two bodies of evidence that lead scientists to believe the levels of dietary supplementation recommended for evening primrose oil and gamma-linolenic acid are safe. The first originates from extrapolations based on the naturally occurring levels of gamma-linolenic acid human infants consume in mature human milk. Research published in the *American Journal of Clinical Nutrition* has shown that each litre of human milk contains between 100 and 400mg of gamma-linolenic acid and its metabolic derivative, dihomo-gamma-linolenic acid. Experts in the use of essential fatty acids point out that if a 5kg (11 lb) infant drinks a litre of milk a day, it consumes between 20 and 80mg of gamma-linolenic acid for each kilogramme of its weight each day. Using *Efamol* as a standard source of omega-6 essential fatty acids, 80mg of gamma-linolenic acid and dihomo-gamma-linolenic acid is the amount found in two 500mg capsules. Therefore, it is reasonable to believe that a gram of evening primrose oil per kilogramme of body weight is safe. Extrapolating forwards, there is no reason to believe that very high doses of essential fatty acids, for example 60g per day for a 60kg (132 lb) adult, will have adverse effects.

Again, it is worth remembering that essential fatty acids are normal parts of natural foods. If they are consumed in quantities larger than the body requires, they are either burned as energy or stored in fat cells as a future source of energy. However, it is always possible that large enough quantities of any substance found in food (for example: salt, various minerals, vitamins, sugar – even water) may prove to be unhealthy in some cases.

Human trials provide the second – and most impressive – data about the safety of *Efamol* evening primrose oil. For example, in a placebo-controlled study of children suffering from cystic fibrosis, patients were given doses as high as 25ml a day for an entire year, and no specific adverse reaction could be attributed to the administration of evening primrose oil.

There are other brands of high quality evening primrose oil products, but the bulk of the controlled clinical research on omega-6 fatty acids has either been conducted or supported by the manufacturers of *Efamol* supplements. Also, proportions of essential fatty acids contained in these products is highly reliable.

Are there special rules for supplements containing omega-6 fatty acids?

When you begin a course of evening primrose supplements, such as the *Efamol* products, six or more 500mg capsules should be taken per day. These can be spread out over two or three meals; but carefully read the packaging of the product you select to make sure it agrees with this advice.

Be prepared to continue taking the supplement for at least four months. Remember that time will be needed to incorporate the essential fatty acids into the cells of your body. As a standard recommendation, begin taking 3g (3,000mg) per day. This dose can be divided, and 1,000mg may be taken before each meal. (Petite women may find beginning with 2,000mg per day satisfactory). Continue this dose for at least a month, then you may wish to reduce your intake to 2,000mg, and after three months a maintenance dose of 500mg per day should care for your basic requirements. During periods of illness or stress you may find a higher dose beneficial for a time.

How should I use essential fatty acid supplements?

Remember that essential fatty acids are natural components of food. Unlike many artificially created pharmaceuticals which need to be taken on an empty stomach to maximize their absorption into the body, essential fatty acid supplements should be taken as part of a normal meal. The natural processes of digestion will release the essential fatty acids into your blood-stream along with other nutrients required for their metabolism.

How does gamma-linolenic acid work?

The therapeutic effects of gamma-linolenic acid, and the other omega-6 fatty acids derived from its metabolism, result from:

- their capacity to alter, or 'modulate' cell membranes,
- their active role in the synthesis and transport of cholesterol,
- their ability to influence the water permeability of the skin and, possibly, tissues in the gastrointestinal system, and . . .
- their regulator capacity when incorporated into molecules of short-lived hormone-like molecules collectively known as eicosanoides.

Are there any side-effects from evening primrose oil?

Some people experience soft stools and/or slight nausea when they first include evening primrose oil in their diet. However, both of these are symptoms one would expect if there was an increase in the quantity of any oil consumed. A few people also experience headaches which have been shown to start and stop when they use evening primrose oil. The body quickly adjusts, however.

Do gamma-linolenic acid supplements work better if I take other supplements as well?

The enzymes involved in the metabolism of linoleic and gamma-linolenic acid require certain minerals and vitamins. These include the metals magnesium, zinc and calcium. Clinical research has also demonstrated a similar requirement for several vitamins, including vitamin C, pyridoxine and biotin.

Some gamma-linolenic acid products are designed to meet specific health requirements, and are packaged to include both essential fatty acids and an appropriate mix of minerals and/or vitamins. *Efacal* is an example. An over-the-counter product in the same family as *Efamol*, *Efacal* was created to help combat the crippling disease, osteoporosis, and therefore contains a balanced combination of evening primrose oil, fish oil and calcium. Tests have shown *Efacal*, taken in combination with certain lifestyle changes (no cigarettes, reduced alcohol consumption, and regular weight-bearing exercise) is an effective way to help control this degenerative illness.

Is it safe to take essential fatty acid supplements for a long period of time?

There is no scientific evidence of side-effects from long-term use of omega-3 and omega-6 fatty acids. This may not be true for all food supplements, however, and all products should be checked for their safety.

Food supplements containing oils should never be used if there is any chance they have become rancid. Read the label carefully and observe the 'Use-by' information.

Diet supplements containing essential fatty acids are fats. Will I gain weight?

Not unless you begin taking quantities of supplements far in excess of those recommended. The number of calories contained in a single supplement capsule is very small.

How much evening primrose oil should I take if I want to prevent illness?

This depends on the product you choose. Suppliers of *Efamol* suggest beginning with six 500mg capsules of evening primrose oil a day for a period of three months. After that, the amount should be reduced to one 500mg capsule per day.

Over the long term, it is difficult to reap benefit from essential fatty acid supplements if the quantity taken is too low, or if the period allowed for them to have an effect is too short. Unlike medications, food supplements work as new building materials for the life-processes carried out by the body's cells to rebuild and replace damaged tissues. This takes time.

Beyond that, it is impossible to prescribe universal rules. Every person's body is different. In general, however, it is suggested that gamma-linolenic acid supplements should be used as long as an individual feels they are receiving benefit.

How much should I take if I have a medical problem?

The answer to this question depends on the problem. As an example, experience working with women suffering from PMS and related breast pain has demonstrated good results with 250-500mg of gamma-linolenic acid a day. If *Efamol* evening primrose oil is used as the source of gamma-linolenic acid, 6-12 capsules (500mg each) per day should have a positive effect. This amount should be continued for a period of up to four months, and then be reduced to one 500mg capsule per day.

Much larger quantities, however, may be needed in certain severe illnesses. As examples, cases of diabetes, inflammatory disease, cancer, and in persons who consumed a diet containing large amounts of saturated fats for a considerable period of time, between 1 and 10g of gamma-linolenic acid per day may be needed. Research suggests 1-2g/day of gamma-linolenic acid may be most effective in the treatment of cardiovascular disease and inflammatory illnesses. In cases of cancer, in which cells are dividing rapidly, 5-15g of gamma-linolenic acid may be needed per day.

It is hoped that current research will provide more specific answers to these questions before the end of the decade.

How do I know if the essential fatty acid supplements are having an effect?

You will see an improvement in your symptoms. Many people using essential fatty acid supplements, but particularly those taking supplements containing evening primrose oil, find other benefits as well. For example, you may use an essential fatty acid supplement for PMS and find that your nails are less likely to break or peel.

If my symptoms improve, how long should I continue taking the supplement, and how much should I take?

This depends on the supplement you are using and your symptoms, but as a general rule, after three months you can cut down the quantity of supplement you take by two-thirds. Instead of taking 3000mg of evening primrose oil each day, cut back to 1000mg. Monitor your symptoms, however, to make certain this amount of essential fatty acids maintains you. If symptoms become worse, increase the amount you take until you see improvement.

Research suggests that a trial period of three to four months is necessary before any significant change can be observed, because the composition of cell membranes is slow to modify. As this rate of change varies from tissue to tissue, weeks – or even months – may pass before a major difference in the proportions of membrane structural elements is significant. Therefore, treatment with gamma-linolenic acid should continue for a considerable period of time.

That can be expensive

Unfortunately, essential fatty acids supplements are expensive. Look for a reputable manufacturer that sells in bulk. This may be identified by reading the material supplied with the product or writing to the company for information. You can also seek advice from your chemist. But, do remember to use supplements provided by a reputable company; don't be tempted by prices that look too good to be true.

Which brands should I buy, and how can I tell the products apart?

The market seems to be flooded with new brands of food supplements everyday. While there are no set rules, give priority to brands that have been around for some time, and are sold by reputable chemists and good health food stores. Your chemist or health food store can be a valuable source of information on a number of nutritional matters, including the choice of diet supplements. Also, see if the packaging includes a help-line, or addresses from which you can obtain additional help. Call or write, and along with your questions concerning your own needs, ask whether or not the advice they give is based on their own research, or information in the literature.

Always check the dates on the packaging to make sure you are buying a fresh product.

It may be interesting to ask whether the company producing the product you choose conducts its own medical research, or depends on data produced by others. Scotia Holdings Plc, manufacturers of *Efamol* products, are a benchmark company in this regard. They support research worldwide, and develop new products based on research conducted by scientists working in independent laboratories around the world. The exact composition of their products is closely monitored to assure therapeutic consistency. The care Scotia Pharmaceuticals takes in maintaining the quality of its products extends to their choice of the specific evening primrose plant they grow to produce the seeds from which they extract the oil they sell.

How should I care for food supplements containing omega-3 and omega-6 fatty acids?

The number of double bonds in the structure of essential fatty acids makes them vulnerable to oxidation, so take the product 'use-by' date seriously. Also, remember to keep your food supplements in a cool place away from direct sunlight. If you live in a warm climate, store them in the refrigerator.

Do essential fatty acids block the effects of, or interact adversely, with any prescribed drugs?

There is no proof that essential fatty acids adversely interact with prescribed drugs, with one important exception. Some research has suggested an interaction between gamma-linolenic acid and phenothiazines, used for the treatment of schizophrenics, which may cause an epileptic seizure. Although this link has not been fully established, *schizophrenics should not be treated with essential fatty acids and gamma-linolenic acid compounds without medical supervision.*

Do any prescribed drugs block the effects of essential fatty acids?

Yes, there is evidence that this can happen. However, when an interaction between a prescribed drug and gamma-linolenic acid, or one of its metabolites, takes place, the therapeutic value of the drug is not changed, but the biological activity of gamma-linolenic acid is hindered. Research is under way to better define these interactions. For example, patients treated with beta-blockers for heart or circulatory conditions may experience a reduced therapeutic result from the gamma-linolenic acid they take as a food supplement. Such an effect can be expected because beta-blockers reduce levels of an important metabolic compound, called Cyclic AMP, in the body. PGE1, the prostaglandin produced as a metabolite of gamma-linolenic acid, interacts with Cyclic AMP, and if levels of Cyclic-AMP are low, the effects of PGE1 will be reduced.

Scientists have also postulated an interaction between steroid drugs, NSAIDs, and two metabolites of gamma-linolenic acid: dihomo-gamma-linolenic and arachidonic acids. Some of these interactions may be beneficial, others may have negative effects. For example, steroids may block the release of arachidonic acid from cell membranes, thus reducing the concentration of harmful tissue substances known as eicosanoids. At the same time, steroids may block the release of dihomo-gamma-linolenic acid, thus reducing the concentration of this important substance available for various cell functions.

Pain-killing NSAIDs, such as ibuprofen, block the production of the prostaglandins that trigger the transmission of pain signals to the brain, but they also inhibit the conversion of dihomo-gamma-linolenic acid to PGE1.

In that case, do any drugs increase my need for gamma-linolenic acid and its metabolites?

Both steroids and NSAIDs can reduce the therapeutic effect of gamma-linolenic acid by blocking the formation of its metabolites. While there are no real guidelines at the present time, scientific knowledge suggests that an increase in the amount of gamma-linolenic acid consumed as a daily food supplement could be worthwhile.

To repeat a vital point of information: *Is it true that people suffering from schizophrenia should not take evening primrose oil unless they are under a doctor's supervision?*

Yes. Based on strong scientific evidence, people suffering from schizophrenia have a special sensitivity to evening primrose oil. When used appropriately, evening primrose oil may have considerable medical benefits. However, incorrect administration may lead to highly undesirable side-effects.

chapter nine

A SUMMING UP

From the moment of conception until the moment of death, an intimate relationship exists between our bodies and the foods we eat. The well-being of the first is inextricably dependent on the other.

Over the past decade, enormous strides have been made in understanding the genetic and protein links between health and disease. Science has truly entered the age of molecular medicine. Now, medical research is proving the importance of another class of nutrients – the essential fatty acids. This work has been a long time in the coming.

Almost four decades ago, Dr Hugh Sinclair postulated the importance of these fragile molecules in sustaining the human body against the degenerative influences of our modern affluent lifestyle. Despite conflict and scientific scorn at that time, his understanding of the role of essential fatty acids in malignant disease, connective tissue and skin disorders, multiple sclerosis, hypertension and coronary thrombosis are now gaining significant credibility.

If we take Professor Sinclair's theories and their implications to their natural conclusions, clearly changes in our modern diet could help reverse many damaging effects of modern living. The keys to the future health of our children and ourselves do not rest in artificially derived chemical counter-agents to disease, but in learning to balance and use the power implicit in natural substances. If we do not act – and act now – to change the way we choose the foods we eat, we are leaving ourselves and future generations open to significant risk. Understanding how we should incorporate essential fatty acids into our daily lives can help change the health status of both the individual, and of society as a whole.

GLOSSARY

acne: Several types of chronic skin disorders in which inflammation involves the hair follicles and the sebaceous glands of the skin.

ageing: Mental and physical changes that occur with the passing of time. The chemical processes controlling the rate of ageing are not well understood, but it is known that free radicals can oxidize molecules in the body's cells, thereby increasing the rate at which tissues, such as skin and the lens of the eye, lose vitality and show signs of degeneration. Some scientists believe antioxidants help slow certain ageing processes by blocking the oxidation by free radicals of essential fatty acids and other susceptible molecules.

AIDS: The complex mix of illnesses and symptoms associated with the Acquired Immune Deficiency Syndrome, which may occur following infection by the HIV virus.

alpha-tocopherol: (see vitamin E)

amino acids: The end-products of the breakdown of proteins during digestion. The basic building blocks of proteins and, therefore, important materials needed for growth, tissue repair and other biological functions. Amino acids take many forms, most of which can be manufactured in the body through processes changing the structure of other amino acids. There are, however, a few of these protein building blocks which must be obtained from the diet. These are called 'essential amino acids'.

antioxidant: Any substance that can interact with free radicals and block their capacity to oxidize other materials. Many antioxidants have been created in the laboratory for use in commercial chemical processes. BHT is an example. However, natural antioxidants are the best choices for blocking unwanted free radical activity in the human body. Vitamin E and vitamin C are the most powerful natural antioxidants; and provitamin A (beta-carotene) is also thought to be effective.

aorta: The primary artery of the body, which leads directly from the heart; its branches and their subdivisions carry oxygen throughout the body.

atherosclerosis: A degenerative disease associated with high levels of saturated fat in the diet, in which cholesterol-rich deposits, called plaques, form on the inner lining and muscle of arteries. As these abnormal areas develop, they weaken the arterial wall, and gradually restrict the size of the lumen through which blood flows. These changes increase the danger of the rupture of the artery wall and high blood pressure. Plaques may break free and block the flow of blood in another location.

Several decades ago, atherosclerosis was found in older individuals, and was thought to be a consequence of ageing. Now, autopsy results demonstrate this condition even in young children.

atom: The smallest particle of an element that can take part in a chemical reaction. Atoms combine to form molecules. Each atom consists of several parts, including a central core, called a nucleus which carries a positive electrical charge, and much smaller bits of matter, called electrons, each of which carries a negative charge. When a molecule loses an electron, changes occur in its capacity to interact with other molecules – this altered structure is called a free radical. Because free radicals pull electrons from other molecules to replace those they have lost, each one exists for a very short period.

atopic eczema: Chronic inflammation of the skin characterized by scaling, redness, itchiness and crusting. The condition may be associated with a family tendency towards allergies.

beta blockers: Drugs that slow the heart rate by blocking certain chemical reactions at nerve endings in cardiac tissue.

BHT: Butylated hydroxytoluene. A synthetic antioxidant used to reduce rancidity in food caused by the oxidation of polyunsaturated fatty acids.

borage (starflower): A herb which grows wild around the Mediterranean Sea. Its blue flowers and leaves have been used for centuries to treat various physical complaints, and in beverages, pot-pourri, and salads. Its seeds are a rich source of essential fatty acids, and contain more than twice the amount of gamma-linolenic acid found in oil from the seeds of the evening primrose. Recent scientific evidence suggests, however, that certain other fatty acids produced in borage seeds may stimulate blood platelets to aggregate, or clot.

cancer: A group of diseases characterized by an uncontrolled growth of abnormal cells.

carbohydrate: Starchy substances in food which, after digestion, provides the body's primary source of energy in the form of the simple sugar, glucose. If all of the energy supplied by carbohydrates is not used, it will be stored as fat.

cardiovascular disease: Any disorder of the heart, blood vessels (vascular system), or circulation of the blood.

atherosclerosis: see above

heart attack (myocardial infarction): The sudden death of part of the heart's muscle owing to oxygen starvation. One cause is a blood clot, or fatty plaque, blocking an artery feeding the heart muscle.

heart failure: As the heart muscle ages, or is attacked by degenerative disease, it may lose its ability to pump hard enough to fully circulate the blood around the body. This leads to stagnation of the blood and the accumulation of fluid in certain tissues. The symptoms of heart failure differ, depending on the side of the heart most seriously damaged.

carotene: An orange pigment found in yellow and red vegetables, including carrots and tomatoes, and green leafy vegetables. Most of the carotene absorbed by the intestinal wall is converted into Vitamin A.

beta-carotene: A specific form of carotene that is a highly effective natural antioxidant.

cataract: A clouding of the eye lens that may lead to blindness. Cataracts are caused by injury, metabolic diseases such as diabetes mellitus, and some of the processes of ageing. Medical research suggests that free radical damage is a cause of this condition, and may be controlled by increasing the dietary intake of antioxidants.

cell: The smallest functioning unit in the body. The human body consists of billions of cells, working and interacting together to accomplish all of the chemical activities necessary for life.

cell membrane: The double-layer structure consisting of protein and fatty substances which encase the internal matter of a cell, and forms boundaries around specific areas of intense chemical activity. Examples are the mitochondria and Golgi body. Essential Fatty Acids form an important part of cell membranes.

cholesterol: A form of fatty substance in the body which is important in the structure of cell membranes, the formation of steroid hormones, the formation of bile salts, and in the transport of fatty acids through the bloodstream to the body's cells. Most cholesterol in the body is manufactured by the liver. High cholesterol levels have been associated with an increased chance of cardiovascular disease; particularly atherosclerosis.

HDL (high-density lipoprotein) cholesterol: A protein-rich form of cholesterol carried in the blood, which seems to protect against arterial and heart disease.

LDL (low density lipoprotein) cholesterol: A low-protein form of blood cholesterol which has been linked with the risk of arterial and heart disease.

chronic degenerative diseases: Illnesses associated with the process of ageing and deterioration of body tissues. People in western societies are more at risk from these conditions than those living in less affluent circumstances. Examples include coronary heart disease, arthritis, cataracts, and osteoporosis.

clinical trial: A research experiment designed to test the therapeutic, protective, or diagnostic capacity of a substance or procedure. There are four levels of clinical trials:

Phase I trials: A new drug is tested on healthy volunteers to determine its safety, the behaviour of the substance in the body, and to establish dosage.

Phase II trials: This is a complex stage of testing in which medical scientists use the new drug on volunteer patients to determine effective dosages, and whether or not the drug may interact with any other medication. Phase II trials are very carefully designed, and are usually based on placebo-controlled investigations.

Phase III trials: This is the pre-marketing phase of drug testing, involving use of the new substance in routine clinical practice. Both the safety and effectiveness of the drug are carefully assessed. Phase I trials through Phase III trials are necessary before a product can be licensed for general use. Because so many tests are required, it usually takes years (as much as a decade) before a new drug is available to the entire population of patients.

Phase IV trials: These are the on-going clinical investigations which take place after a drug has reached the market.

coronary artery disease: Damage to the heart caused by blockage or diminished flow of blood to its muscle because of blood clots and/or obstruction from atherosclerotic plaque.

dermatitis: Inflammation of the skin characterized by itching, roughness, and eruptions of unknown cause. In many cases, these reactions may be associated with allergic reactions, including hay fever.

diabetes mellitus: An illness characterized by the abnormal metabolism of blood sugar caused by a reduced production of the hormone insulin by the pancreas.

diabetic neuropathy: The biochemical consequences of diabetes may result in long-term degeneration of the peripheral nerves, causing pain or loss of sensation.

diet: A combination of all of the foods and fluids consumed. The word 'diet' is also used to describe a prescribed intake of foods and fluids for therapeutic or weight-loss purposes.

digestion: The group of physical and chemical processes which lead to the breakdown of the foods and fluids we eat into their fundamental units. Proteins are broken down into amino acids, carbohydrates into glucose, and fats into fatty acids, cholesterol, and other complex lipids. The products of digestion are used in the metabolic processes of the body necessary for growth, energy, repair, and so on.

DNA: deoxyribonucleic acid. The double-helix molecule, primarily found in the nucleus of cells, which contains the genetic code to the unique structures and functions of the individual.

eczema: A common name for chronic and acute inflammation and breakdown of the skin leading to itching, blistering and scaling. Eczema is sometimes referred to as 'dermatitis'.

atopic eczema: see above

eicosanoids: Short-lived regulatory substances in the body which are derived from arachidonic acid. These highly active molecules serve as short-range communicators between cells. Both prostaglandins and leukotriens are eicosanoids, derived from arachidonic acid.

electron: A sub-atomic particle which carries a negative charge, and circles the nucleus of an atom, which carries a positive charge. When electrons are missing from an atom, or occur in excess, a free radical is formed.

element: Any one of the basic natural substances which form all matter on earth. A substance composed of only one type of atom.

enzymes: A large family of highly specific proteins which are manufactured in the body's cells. Enzymes are organic catalysts which accelerate chemical changes in other substances.

epidermis: The external, protective skin covering the body.

epidemiology: The scientific study of diseases within populations.

epithelium: A continuous layer of cells covering all surfaces of the body – cutaneous, mucous, and serous. The characteristics of these cells vary according to their location. They are important because they form boundaries between organs and between other distinct functioning parts.

evening primrose: An ancient plant originating in North America, but now growing throughout Europe. Oil from the seeds of the evening primrose is rich in gamma-linolenic acid, which has been shown to have important biological properties. Although other seed oils contain higher percentages of gamma-linolenic acid, evening primrose oil contains fewer extraneous fatty acids, some of which may prove to have a toxic effect.

fat: (see lipids) A greasy substance found in animals and some plants which is rich in energy. Without fats of various types, the body could not function properly. By weight, fats make up 10 per cent of the normal human body.

fatty acid: The prevalent form of fat in the human body, usually found attached to another molecule; for example, in triglycerides – the most common form of fat in the body – three fatty acid molecules attach to one molecule of glycerol. Fatty acids consist of a string of carbon atoms which end in a chemical 'hook', called a carboxyl group. This 'hook' attaches the fatty acid to the glycerol molecule, to a protein, or to a molecule of cholesterol.

cis-*fatty acids:* The natural, biologically active molecular form of unsaturated fatty acids. In this form, the unsaturated, double-bonds of the molecule are capable of rapid interaction with other molecules. They are easily oxidized, and may cause food to become rancid.

Essential fatty acid: Strictly speaking, a specific group of fatty acids which the human body cannot manufacture, and includes only linoleic acid (an omega-6 fatty acid) and alpha-linolenic acid (an omega-3 fatty acid). However, this classification is often extended to include fatty acids manufactured by the body from this pair of fatty acids.

Monounsaturated fatty acid: A fatty acid with only one double bond in its structure. Oleic acid is the most common form of natural monounsaturated fatty acid. Particularly high concentrations are found in olive oil.

Polyunsaturated fatty acid: A fatty acid with two or more double bonds in its carbon chain. Linoleic acid is an example of an essential fatty acid with two double bonds.

gamma-linolenic acid (GLA): A biologically significant metabolite of linoleic acid, which is necessary for a number of important cellular functions. Certain plant oils, including that from evening primrose and borage seeds contain large quantities of this essential fatty acid.

linoleic acid (LA): An unsaturated fatty acid essential for normal growth and health. The enzyme which transforms this fatty acid into the more biologically active GLA is easily blocked by a number of lifestyle and environmental factors.

omega-3 fatty acids (also called n-3 fatty acids): A series of fatty acids in which an unsaturated double bond occurs at the n-3 position in its carbon chain. All omega-3 fatty acids are derived from alpha-linolenic acid.

omega-6 fatty acids (also called n-6 fatty acids): A series of fatty acids in which an unsaturated double bond occurs at the n-6 position in its carbon chain. All omega-6 fatty acids derive from linoleic acid.

saturated fatty acids: Fatty acids in which the carbon chain contains no double-bonds. Fats rich in saturated fatty acids harden when chilled.

trans-*fatty acids:* An abnormal, biologically inactivated molecular form of unsaturated fatty acid, including essential fatty acids. Because the body cannot access the critical unsaturated parts of these molecules for special purposes – such as the manufacture of prostaglandins – they are used for energy and metabolized in much the same way as saturated fats. Many processes used in the manufacture of foods change unsaturated fatty acids from the *cis-* to *trans-* form as a means of reducing the risk of products becoming rancid through oxidation.

fibre (dietary): Various forms of complex plant carbohydrate which cannot be broken down and digested by the human body as a source of energy. Dietary fibre is important as bulk.

fibrocystic breast disease: A benign disease resulting in the formation of painful, lumpy tissue in the breast. However, if any lumps are found in the breasts, medical advice should be sought (see: mastalgia).

fish oils: (see marine oil) Rich sources of omega-3 fatty acids. These substances are stored in the tissues of fish which feed on marine plants which produce these fatty acids.

free radical: A molecule in which negatively charged electrons and positively charged protons are out of balance; i.e. there is one too many or one too few electrons circling its positively charged nucleus. Free radicals are highly unstable, and will destroy other molecules in their environment to correct their electrical balance. For example, free radicals containing too few electrons will 'grab' electrons from other molecules.

gerontology: The scientific study of the ageing process and its related problems.

glucose: The simple form of carbohydrate, which is the primary source of energy in living things.

glycogen: The form of carbohydrate (glucose molecules) stored in animal tissues.

gynaecology: The medical speciality concerning the female reproductive system.

heart attack: See cardiovascular disease.

heart failure: See cardiovascular disease.

hormones: A group of chemical substances produced by specific organs in the body, which are carried by the bloodstream to other tissues and organs where they cause metabolic changes.

hydroxyl radical: A powerful form of free radical consisting of an oxygen atom and a hydrogen atom, paired with only one electron.

hyperkinesis: Another name for hyperactivity. Behavioural patterns of children who have difficulty concentrating and are constantly overactive.

immune system: The combination of cells and biological activities in the body which work together to fight invasion by bacteria, viruses and fungi. The immune system is also important in the control of the spread of cancer cells, and may be responsible for allergic reactions and rejection of transplanted organs.

inflammation: A specific series of biological and chemical processes which, following injury or disease, cause blood vessels and the surrounding tissue in an affected area to redden, swell, become hot, and cause pain. White blood cells usually accumulate in inflamed tissue to help destroy invading infection and/or repair damaged tissues. Inflammation is a vital part of the body's response to attack by external forces.

ion: An electrically charged atom or molecule formed when an electron is lost or gained. An atom or molecule out of 'electrical balance'.

irritable bowel syndrome (IBS): A condition, characterized by a combination of abdominal pain, constipation and/or looseness of the bowels, for which no specific organic cause can be identified. In many cases, this condition is worse before the start of menstruation, and may be related to the level of certain prostaglandins.

kidney stone: An abnormal lump of mineral salts – called a urinary calculus – formed in the kidney from the precipitation of calcium, phosphate and magnesium. Similar stones may form in the ureters and urinary bladder.

leukotrienes: Hormone-like molecules, derived from the essential fatty acid arachidonic acid, which have been shown to play roles in tissue inflammation and allergic reactions.

lipids: A general term describing any substance which is insoluble in water, but soluble in an organic solvent – such as chloroform or ether. Lipids include fatty acids, cholesterol, steroids, phospholipids, triglycerides and waxes.

liver: The largest organ in the human body, and the furnace of metabolic activity. Among its many functions, the liver produces cholesterol and aids in the mobilization of fats.

marine oils: Oils extracted from fish, which are rich in omega-3 fatty acids. Examples are cod liver oil, salmon oil, and halibut liver oil. The latter should be used with caution, as it contains high levels of vitamin D. Quantities of Vitamin D in excess of need are stored in the liver, and may cause abnormal deposits of calcium in the body's tissues.

mastalgia: Breast pain, often experienced in the days preceding menstruation. Mastalgia is a common medical condition and can, at time, be severe.

Mediterranean Diet: A name used to describe a diet rich in complex carbohydrates – such as pasta – fresh vegetables and fruits. Like the favourite foods of people living around the

Mediterranean, this diet contains ample quantities of olive oil, but is low in saturated fats. Population research indicates a comparatively low risk of heart attack and cancer among people normally living on this combination of foods.

meta-analysis: A method of data analysis involving the accumulation and combined analysis of information from a number of research studies concerning a specific question – for example, what is the relationship between dietary fat and heart disease. Meta-analysis is sometimes criticized because of variability introduced by collectively studying data from a number of different investigations. The studies grouped together for analysis may have taken place over one or more decades, and would have used several different methods of investigation and data collection. However, others believe the massive amount of information that can be combined in meta-analysis smooths out any inconsistency.

metabolism: A group of chemical processes in the body which break down complex substances (catabolism), such as sugars and fats, for use as energy or for use in the construction of new compounds (anabolism). The results of metabolism include tissue repair, growth, and energy production.

micronutrients: Substances in foods which are necessary in very small quantities for normal growth and good health. These include vitamins, trace elements, and certain other substances, including the essential fatty acids.

minerals: In the context of nutrition, minerals are those chemical elements which must be present in the diet for good health. Some, such as calcium and potassium, are needed in large quantities. Others known as 'trace elements', including selenium and zinc, are needed in very small quantities, but are absolutely essential for normal life processes to continue.

mitochondria: Highly specialized membrane structures within the substance of cells These structures are the cell's key source of energy and are responsible for many of the body's complex biochemical activities. Lipids, especially essential fatty acids, form a vital part of their membrane structure.

mucosa: The layer of epithelial cells lining certain body cavities, including the digestive tract, the genital passages, and the respiratory tract. Essential fatty acids in the membranes of these cells are especially important as regulators of molecules which flow into and out of the body.

molecule: The smallest unit, or particle, of a substance containing two or more atoms, which retain the chemical properties of the substance.

multiple sclerosis (MS): A progressive degenerative disease of the fatty, myelin coating of nerve fibres in the spinal cord and brain. Symptoms vary according to where the lesions occur.

NSAIDs: Non-steroidal anti-inflammatory drugs, for example aspirin and ibuprofen, used to suppress pain and inflammation. Strong evidence indicates that NSAIDs inhibit the production of prostaglandins in the gastric mucosa, thus increasing the chance of ulcer formation.

nutrition: The scientific study of food and water requirements for normal growth and good health. 'Good Nutrition' is a term used to describe an appropriate dietary balance of foods and fluids.

oleic acid: An unsaturated fatty acid, containing only one double bond in its carbon chain. Oleic acid is the most abundant and widely distributed fatty acid in nature. It is found in high quantities in olive oil.

organ: Any part of the body responsible for a specific function. For example, the heart is the organ responsible for pumping blood round the body.

osteoporosis: Loss of bone tissue associated with a reduction in the quantity of protein supporting its structure. Osteoporosis is a natural consequence of ageing. However, in post-menopausal women, elderly men, and people consuming diets deficient in calcium, the condition may lead to debilitating spontaneous fractures of the bone.

oxidation: A chemical reaction in which a molecule combines with an oxygen molecule and loses one or more electrons to it. Free radicals (see above) oxidize other molecules, including unsaturated fatty acids. Some forms of oxidation are important steps in normal biological activity. However, excessive oxidation can result in abnormal biological activity and tissue damage.

pancreas: A large glandular organ located in the upper abdomen which secretes insulin – a hormone important in carbohydrate metabolism – and pancreatic juices, which contain enzymes important in fat and protein metabolism.

phospholipid: A fat molecule containing one or more atoms of phosphorous. There are several important families of phospholipids found in tissues throughout the body. Lecithin, for example, is a phospholipid found in high concentrations in the protective covering, known as the myelin sheath, around nerves.

placebos: Preparations used in controlled clinical studies which do not have any specific pharmacological purpose or activity.

plant oils: Oils extracted from plant seeds and fruits parts (such as the meaty part of olives). These have been shown to have value as sources of essential fatty acids.

plaque (arterial): The name given to fatty patches (areas of atherosclerosis) on the inner walls of arteries. These cholesterol-rich deposits invade, and thereby weaken, arterial walls.

premenstrual syndrome (PMS): A combination of physical and mental changes experienced by many women a week or more before the start of menstruation. Certain prostaglandins, Vitamin E and B-complex vitamins have been demonstrated to reduce symptoms in a percentage of cases. Gamma-linolenic acid has been found to reduce symptoms.

prostaglandin: A form of local hormone, or cell regulator, containing an essential fatty acid. Specific prostaglandins have been shown to lower blood-pressure, stimulate contraction of the uterus and change the 'stickiness' of blood platelets. Certain prostaglandins cause inflammation.

prospective research: Experimental trials in which the conditions of the investigation are defined before the research is begun. Variables which may influence the results are controlled as tightly as possible.

protein: A basic nutritional requirement for growth and health. Proteins are obtained from both plant and animal sources. Protein in foods is broken down during digestion into small units known as amino acids. Following release into the bloodstream, these simple building blocks are reconstituted into the complex protein chains found in the muscles and other structures of the body.

provitamin: A substance in food which the body uses as the foundation for building a vitamin. For example, the body uses beta-carotene to manufacture vitamin A.

rancid: The distinctive foul taste and smell produced when the unsaturated fatty acids in foods are oxidized. Rancid foods are highly undesirable. To prolong the shelf-life of their merchandise, food manufacturers either add antioxidant to foods, or change the structure of fat molecules to decrease their susceptibility to oxidation. In the latter case, *cis-* fatty acids are often transformed into the *trans-* configuration.

relative deficiency: Through starvation, illness, or during prolonged dieting, it is possible to consume adequate amounts of essential nutrients to avoid specific deficiency diseases, such as scurvy, but not enough to avoid degenerative diseases.

RNA (ribonucleic acid): A form of genetic material that occurs both inside and outside the cell nucleus.

schizophrenia: The classification for a number of disabling mental illnesses which involve bizarre behaviour, thinking and emotional response to life circumstances. Patients known to be suffering from schizophrenia should not take evening primrose oil, or other dietary supplements containing essential fatty acids, unless it is administered under medical supervision.

scurvy: A serious illness, involving connective tissues, which results from a deficiency of vitamin C. Scurvy is characterized by abnormal bleeding of the gums, loosening of teeth, and bleeding into the muscles.

selenium: One of the trace elements which has been shown to 'help' antioxidants deactivate free radicals. Selenium is essential in small amounts for a number of biological functions. However, if taken in excess, it can be toxic.

serous membrane: The thin layer of epithelial cells which forms a continuous lining over all of the organs of the closed cavities of the body. They secrete a thin fluid which serves as a lubricant when organs or structural parts move against one another – for example, the articulation within joints and the movement of the lungs within the rib-cage.

serum: The clear fluid which separates from blood when it clots.

serum lipids: Fats which circulate in the serum portion of the blood. Raised serum lipid levels are associated with the development of coronary disease.

starflower: See borage.

thrombosis: A blood clot in an artery or vein.

tissue: A collection of cells, all of which have a common purpose. Groups of 'tissue' form an 'organ'.

tocopherol: The first name given to vitamin E. However, it is now a generic term for vitamin E and related compounds.

alpha-tocopherol: The biologically active form of tocopherol, and is the true form of vitamin E. Alpha-tocopherol is an oily substance which may be obtained from wheatgerm oil, or made by synthetic means. A powerful natural antioxidant which protects fats.

triglyceride: A fat consisting of three fatty acid molecules attached to a molecule of glycerol. Triglycerides are the main form of fats stored in the body, and serve as an energy reserve.

vitamins: A group of complex substances which cannot be manufactured in the body, but are necessary in small amounts for normal health and to fight illness. Absence of any of these substances will lead to a deficiency disease. For example, over time, a diet lacking vitamin C will result in the illness, scurvy.

There are two types of vitamins: water-soluble (vitamin C, for example) and fat-soluble (vitamins A, D, E and K). Good sources of dietary fat are required for proper absorption of the fat-soluble vitamins.

vitamin E: A fat-soluble, powerful natural antioxidant found in certain plant oils (see tocopherol). Like other fat-soluble vitamins, E is stored in the fatty tissues of the body and in the liver, and daily intake may not be necessary.

vitamin C: A water-soluble vitamin that acts as a powerful antioxidant. Like other water-soluble vitamins, C is removed quickly from the body and excess is excreted in the urine. Top-ups are therefore necessary through either the diet or supplements.

FAT COMPOSITION
OF SELECTED FOODS

A few words about reading tables

The following tables are provided to give you some ideas about which foods are rich in the nurtients you want to include in your diet, such as polyunsaturated fatty acids and natural antioxidants. However, before using this or any other information concerning the composition of foods, remember that there are no absolutes.

Numbers on a page may tell you that 100g of pork chops have 'x' grams of saturated fat and 'y' grams of unsaturates, but the actual amount on your plate may vary. The size of your portion, how the food was prepared, and even what animals were given to eat before they were slaughtered, will influence the nutrients on your dinner table. While it is true that reputable scientists publish data based on pooled information from a number of samples, these specimens may not represent what you are about to eat.

Even the soil in which crops are grown may influence which nutrients are available in food. For example, according to McCance and Widdowson's *The Composition of Foods, 5th Edition*, which is the source for these tables, 100g of 'old' potatoes, baked and served in their skins, will provide about 2 micrograms (a microgram is one millionth of a gram) of selenium. However, that figure depends on where the potatoes were grown. Some agricultural areas produce fine vegetables, but because the land may be naturally low in certain minerals – selenium is a case in point – the food grown on that land may contain minimal amounts.

As you look through the tables in this book, notice how cooking methods and age of certain crops – carrots, for example – influence key nutrients.

Table 1: **Dietary sources rich in specific types of fatty acids**

Type of fat	Animal sources	Plant sources
Saturated	Beef Lamb Egg yolk Dairy products Poultry	Palm oil Coconut oil
Monounsaturated		Olive oil Peanut oil Rapeseed oil
Polyunsaturated	Oily fish, including: salmon herring anchovies mackerel	Corn oil Cottonseed oil Safflower oil Soya oil Sunflower oil Wheatgerm oil

Table 2: **Composition of fats in popular meats (contained in 100g servings)**

Food	kcal (1)	Total fat grams (2)	Sat fat grams (1)	Mono unsat grams (1)	Poly unsat grams (1)	Sat fat % (1)	Mono unsat % (3)	Poly unsa % (3
Bacon: gammon lean, grilled	172	5.2	1.9	2.2	0.5	41.3	47.8	10.9
Ham: canned	120	5.1	1.9	2.1	0.6	41.3	45.7	13
Beef: rump grilled	218	12.1	5.2	5.8	0.5	45.2	50.4	4.3
Beef: sirloin roast	284	20.1	9.0	10.2	0.9	44.8	50.7	4.5
Lamb: chops grilled	355	29.0	14.4	11.2	1.4	53.3	41.5	5.2
Lamb: leg roast	266	17.9	8.9	6.9	0.9	53.3	41.3	5.4

Food	kcal (1)	Total fat grams (2)	Sat fat grams (1)	Mono unsat grams (1)	Poly unsat grams (1)	Sat fat % (1)	Mono unsat % (3)	Poly unsat % (3)
Pork: chops grilled	332	24.2	9	9.8	3.6	40.2	43.8	16.1
Pork: leg roast	286	19.8	7.3	8.0	3.0	39.9	43.7	16.4
Chicken roast:								
light meat	142	4.0	1.2	1.9	0.7	31.6	50.0	18.4
dark meat	155	6.9	2.1	3.2	1.2	32.3	49.2	18.5
Duck: roast meat only	189	9.7	2.7	5.3	1.2	29.3	57.6	13.0
Turkey roast:								
light meat	132	1.4	0.4	0.6	0.3	30.8	46.2	23.0
dark meat	148	4.1	1.3	1.7	0.8	34.2	44.7	21.0

1 These data are from *The Composition of Foods, 5th Edition,* and are reproduced with the permission of The Royal Society of Chemistry and the Controller of Her Majesty's Stationery Office.

Figures in this table are based on the analysis of a number of samples. Nevertheless, keep in mind that these are approximations, and amounts and percentages may be influences by a number of factors, including how the meat was prepared.

Note how the amount of fat varies from one type of meat to another. According to this source, 100g of beef (sirloin) roast contains 29g of fat, while the same weight of light meat from turkey contains only 1.4g. Also, note that meats from the same type of animal tend to contain approximately the same proportion of different types of fatty acids. For example, the figures for the lamb chops and roast leg of lamb are very similar, although the chops contain more fat than the roasted meat.

2 Note that the figure for the total grams of fat in each type of food is greater than the sum of the gram weight for specific types of fatty acids reported in the next three columns (Saturated, Monounsaturated and Polyunsaturated). This is because there are types of fats other than fatty acids present. Cholesterol is one example. Another is glycerol, to which fatty acids are bound in triglyceride molecules.

3 These figures are based on the weight of various categories of fatty acids reported in each type of meat. As percentages, they reflect the degree of saturation or unsaturation. Grilled lamb chops, for example, are very high in saturated fatty acids (53.3%). Duck is high in monounsaturated fatty acids (57.6%) and comparatively low in saturated fats (29.3).

***Table 3:* Fatty acid composition of fats and oils per 100g (3)**

Food	Kcal (1)	Sat fat grams/ tbsp (1)	Mono unsat grams/ tbsp (1)	Poly unsat grams/ tbsp (1) (2)	Sat fat grams/ tbsp (2)	Mono unsat grams/ tbsp (2)	Poly unsat grams/ tbsp (2) (3)
Butter	737	54	19.8	2.6	8.1	3.0	0.4
Margarine (veg.)							
hard	739	35.9	33	9.4	5.4	5.0	1.4
soft	739	25.0	31	21.8	3.8	4.7	3.3
Beef drippng	891	54.8	36.7	2.5	8.2	5.5	0.4
Lard	891	40.8	43.8	9.6	6.1	6.6	1.4
Blended veg. oil	899	10.4	35.5	48.2	1.6	5.3	7.2
Coconut oil	899	85.2	6.6	1.7	12.8	1.0	0.3
Corn oil	899	12.7	24.7	57.8	1.9	3.7	8.7
Olive oil	899	14.7	69.2	112.1	2.1	10.4	1.7
Peanut oil	899	18.8	47.8	28.5	2.8	7.1	4.3
Safflower oil	899	10.2	12.6	72.1	1.5	1.9	10.8
Soya oil	899	14.5	23.2	56.5	2.2	3.5	8.5
Sunflower oil	899	11.9	20.2	63	1.8	3.0	9.4
Wheatgerm oil	899	18.8	15.9	60.7	2.8	2.4	9.1

1 These data are from *The Composition of Foods, 5th Edition,* and are reproduced with the permission of The Royal Society of Chemistry and the Controller of Her Majesty's Stationery Office.

2 The figures presented in the first four columns of this table are taken from the source noted above, and represent the amounts of various types of fatty acids found in 100g of specific oils. However, it is often more helpful to know the relative quantities of fatty acids in the volumes of oil we use in everyday meal preparation. For dressing and cooking food, a tablespoon is a convenient measure. Columns 5, 6 and 7 show approximate amounts of types of fatty acids found in a tablespoonful (approximately 15g) of each oil listed. Volume weights of oils vary slightly, so use these figures as a guide, and not absolutes.

3 The figures for polyunsaturates are all inclusive, and no attempt has been made to estimate *cis-* and *trans-* forms of these molecules.

Table 4: **Fats in nuts, seeds and seed casings (per 100g portions)**

Food	Calories	Saturated fat grams	Monounsat fat grams	Polyunsat fat grams
Almonds	612	4.7	34.4	14.2
Brazil nuts	682	16.4	25.8	23.0
Cashew nuts	611	10.1	29.4	9.1
Coconut:				
creamed block	669	59.3	3.9	1.6
Macadamia nuts	748	11.2	60.8	1.6
Peanuts – plain	564	8.2	21.1	14.3
Pecan nuts	689	5.7	42.5	18.7
Pine nuts	688	4.6	19.9	41.1
Sesame seeds	598	8.3	21.7	25.5
Sunflower seeds	581	4.5	9.8	31.0
Walnuts	688	5.6	12.4	47.5
Avocado	190	4.1	12.1	2.2
Olives	103	1.7	5.7	1.3

These data are from *The Composition of Foods, 5th Edition*, and are reproduced with the permission of The Royal Society of Chemistry and the Controller of Her Majesty's Stationery Office.

Table 5: **Fish favourites – grams of fatty acid in 100g servings**

Food	Calories	Saturated fat	Monounsat fat	Polyunsat fat
White fish				
Cod:				
baked	96	0.5	0.2	0.2
fried/oil	199	0.9	5.1	3.7
fried/dripping	199	4.7	3.1	0.2
Haddock:				
steamed	98	0.2	0.1	0.3
fried/oil	160	0.7	3.8	2.8
fried/dripping	160	3.5	2.3	0.1
Oily fish				
Mackerel: fried	188	2.3	5.6	2.3
Herring: fried	234	4.3	6.9	2.5
Herring grilled	199	3.7	5.9	2.1
Salmon:				
steamed	197	2.4	5.5	3.7
smoked	142	0.8	1.9	1.3
canned	155	1.5	3.5	2.4

These data are from *The Composition of Foods, 5th Edition*, and are reproduced with the permission of The Royal Society of Chemistry and the Controller of Her Majesty's Stationery Office.

Table 6: Fatty acid content of selected meat products (100g samples)

Food	Calories	Saturated fat (grams)	Monounsat fat (grams)	Polyunsat fat (grams)
Beefburgers: frozen/fried	264	8	7.8	0.7
Corned beef: canned	217	6.3	4.8	0.3
Luncheon meat: canned	313	9.8	12.4	3.3
Sausage roll (flaky pastry)	477	13.4	15.6	5.3
Steak and kidney pie (individual)	323	8.4	9.7	2.1
Beef curry (retail)	137	3.1	2.5	0.6
Bolognese sauce	145	3.1	4.7	2.6
Chicken curry (without bone)	205	2.2	6	7.5
Lasagna (low fat)	102	1.9	1.4	0.2

These data are from *The Composition of Foods, 5th Edition*, and are reproduced with the permission of The Royal Society of Chemistry and the Controller of Her Majesty's Stationery Office.

FOODS RICH IN
NATURAL ANTIOXIDANTS

DATA in this section are from *The Composition of Foods, 5th Edition*, and are reproduced with the permission of The Royal Society of Chemistry and the Controller of Her Majesty's Stationery Office.

Vitamin C (mg/100g)

Breakfast cereals (commercial brands):

Bran flakes	25
Ready Brek	27
Start	37
Weetos	30

Vegetables (mg/100g)

Beans – French/green (raw)	12
Broccoli (raw)	87
(boiled)	44
Brussels sprouts (raw)	115
(boiled)	60
Cabbage (raw)	49
(boiled)	20
Green peppers (raw)	120
(boiled)	69
Mange-tout (raw)	54
(boiled)	28
Peas (fresh/boiled)	16
Potatoes (new)	16
(old)	11
Spinach (raw)	26
(boiled)	8

Spring greens (raw)	180
(cooked)	77
Sweet potatoes (boiled)	17
Tomatoes (raw)	17

Other (mg/100g)

Parsley (raw)	190
Watercress (raw)	62

Fruit (raw, unless otherwise indicated) (mg/100g)

Apple (raw and peeled)	14
Avocado	6
Blackcurrants	200
Clementines	54
Grapefruit	36
Guava	230
Lemon (whole)	58
Lychees	45
Mangoes	37
Melon (cantaloupe type)	26
Nectarine	37
Oranges	54
Paw-paw	60
Raspberries	32
Strawberries	77
Tangerines	30

Vitamin E

Oils (mg/100g)

Cottonseed	42.8
Olive	5.1
Palm	33.1
Peanut	15.2
Rapeseed	22.2
Safflower	40.7
Soya	16.3
Sunflower	49.2
Wheatgerm	136.7

Nuts (shelled) and Seeds (mg/100g)

Almonds	24.0
Hazelnuts	25.0
Peanuts	10.1
Pine nuts	13.7
Sunflower seeds	37.8

Vegetables and Fruits (mg/100g)

Avocado	3.2
Brussels sprouts	1.0
Leeks	0.8
Spinach (raw)	1.7
Sweet potatoes (raw)	4.6
Tomatoes (raw)	1.2
Watercress	1.5

Carotene (micrograms/100g)

Tip: Carotene give fruits and vegetables a bright orange or red colour. It also deepens the green in certain produce. Use this as a guide when you select fresh foods.

Vegetables (raw, unless otherwise indicated) (micrograms/100g)

Broad beans	225
Runner beans	145
Mange-tout	695
Peas	300
Broccoli	575
Cabbage	385
Carrots (old)	8,115
(young)	5,330
Courgette	610
Curly kale	3,145
Leeks	735
Okra	515
Pumpkin (cooked)	955
Spinach	3,535
Sweet potatoes	3,930

Red pepper (capsicum)	3,840
Tomatoes	640
(purée)	1,300
Watercress	2,520

Fruit (raw) (micrograms/100g)

Apricots	405
Guava	435
Mango	1,800
Melon (cantaloupe-type)	1,000
Passion fruit	750
Paw-paw	810
Plums	295

Other foods (micrograms/100g)

Paprika	36,250
Parsley	4040

(Other herbs and spices that are rich in carotene, but for which there is less specific data, include: chilli powder, rosemary, sage and thyme.)

MEDICAL NEWS IN THE PRESS

Is it useful?

Medical research summarized in the popular press plays a surprisingly important role in our daily lives. But should it? How can we know which claims to take seriously, and which to dismiss with a smile?

Reports of new medical ideas and experiments influence us in several ways. Most obviously, they make eyecatching headlines in newspapers and television programmes, and most of us are hungry for the details. A report covering a miraculous cure for a deadly disease, or a story about a surgical procedure shown to erase the signs of ageing, is quick to attract our attention. We want to read about medical research because we want to be well, look good and live long, productive lives.

This desire to feel and look our best is valuable. It inspires us to accept lifestyle changes that might otherwise be contrary to our nature. Practising safe sex is an example; giving up cigarettes is another. We learn from good medical journalism, and it can literally save lives.

Good medical reporting educates us in ways that make it easier to understand and cope with our own health problems. We often learn about developments in medicine from a newspaper or magazine article before we hear about them from our doctor. A well-presented television programme concerning an open heart operation can reassure a patient facing surgery. Information about self-examination for testicular and breast cancer can help flag problems at an early stage. And, understanding an illness from news items we read about or see on television can help us communicate better with a doctor or therapist.

Unfortunately, not all reports we read, or see on television, are prepared by journalists of the same standard. Experimental data, properly reported in a highly reputable medical journal, may be taken out of context, or not fully reported in the popular press. The final press story may be more dramatic, but it can also mislead members of the public.

There is another, more subtle way reports about medical research influence the way we live. They indirectly change the range of products, particularly food and drink, available to us in stores and supermarkets. Often this is an ideal situation; it provides more resources to help change our lifestyle. In other ways, however, the product manufacturers may benefit more than the public. Manufacturers respond to changes in public health attitudes by amending their line of products to meet public demand. Unfortunately, these expanding product lines, and the advertising used to sell them, can encourage misinterpretation of the facts as presented in the original scientific medical report.

The surge in the number of low-fat and fat-free products on the market has created a major change in product design. For years, scientists have known about the link between high levels of dietary fat and heart disease, and advised people to change their eating habits. Public interest created a demand for low-fat butter substitutes containing polyunsaturated oils. Soon, many alternatives were on the supermarket shelves. Unfortunately, the increasing number of these products, and the resulting advertising to support competition between brands, enhanced their credibility as healthy alternatives to butter. It was not until later that most medical journalists became aware of *trans*-forms of polyunsaturated fatty acids, and the fact that these molecules are created when polyunsaturated oils are changed from a liquid to a solid form during the manufacture of many butter substitutes. It was only then the public learned *trans*-polyunsaturated fats behave like saturated fats in the body, and are just as damaging.

As another example of misuse of scientific data, consider the case of low-fat foods. There is ample research evidence to show that decreasing the amount of fat in our diet reduces the risk of certain killer diseases. However, some media health 'gurus' went so far as to say that very-low-fat-diets, even no-fat diets, are healthy choices. Legitimate health experts know this is not true, but enough members of the public were convinced to create a demand for new, low-fat food products. Manufacturers responded by creating a wide range of products, including fat-free ice cream: high in carbohydrates, but fatless. Regrettably, some people using these products did not appreciate that no-fat is different from no-calories, and have found themselves gaining weight while binging on fat-free foods!

How does medical research get reported? And why can't they get it right the first time?

In all fields of science, knowledge develops one step at a time. Scientists design and conduct experiments based on previously published theories and data, and add to these as new results are verified. Small variations in the way an experiment is carried out, or in the subjects chosen to participate in an investigation, may provide results that are at odds with existing research findings and accepted theories. These are not setbacks, but a source of new ideas in the body of information that fuel future research. The new findings must be re-examined and independently tested by other qualified investigators.

Scientific ideas and theories can be changed by many things; and one is the introduction of a new technology. In the study of dietary fats, for example, the introduction of gas-liquid chromatography (a method used to identify groups of molecules in a substance by measuring their relative rate of separation under controlled conditions of heat and volatility) made it possible for scientists to separate, quantify and identify very small samples of fatty acids, thus opening their eyes to relationships they could previously only guess at. But, equipment is not the only thing that can change in a laboratory. Methods used to analyse research results can also change. One such change, which has profoundly influenced the scientific papers currently being published, is *meta-analysis*.

Meta-analysis involves combining and statistically analysing information from many published research reports in an attempt to remove, or compensate for, any ambiguity in their conclusions. Consider, for example, the work done over the past five decades on heart disease and diet. Results from individual studies do not agree, and considerable contradiction exists.

Many public health statisticians believe that, if enough scientific studies completed over a long period of time can be combined, some differences in experimental design can be smoothed out, and reasons for contradiction can be compensated for. However, meta-analysis also has its detractors, who believe that this means of data analysis only adds confusion, and its results should be read with a certain degree of caution.

Who is right? The experts will argue that one out. For the rest of us, we need to be aware of how fragile the findings of scientific research really are.

All experiments claiming to be *scientific* must be conducted under a strict set of rules, known as the Scientific Method. These rules dictate how questions are formulated, how subjects used in the experiment are selected and controlled, how data are gathered and how results are analysed. Once results have been obtained by these means, they are verified in the same laboratory several times, using the same methods, before a report is written. Through their report, investigators want to convey their findings and ideas to others in their field, and it will be submitted, in the required format and style, for publication in a specific scientific journal well respected in the particular area of research. Before accepting the report for publication, the journal's editorial board will have it reviewed by people recognized as highly expert in the subject covered by the report. This process is known as 'peer review', and most of the time it works very well. If these experts feel the research is in some way flawed, or that its conclusions need further explanation, the journal will send it back to its author, who may choose to respond to these criticisms, or send the report on to another journal for consideration.

The complexity and lengthy nature of peer review prior to publication of research can frustrate the acknowledgement of a new approach to an old problem. It can also delay acceptance of a new theory that runs against the grain of current thinking. Highly controversial ideas and data are sometimes difficult to get published, not because the research that has produced them is flawed, but because other scientists find them difficult to accept.

The peer review control in scientific literature has no parallel in the popular media. This is unfortunate, because journalists working for the popular press interpret scientific findings for the public. In the end, our understanding of a scientific investigation is no better than the quality of the journalist who writes the articles we read with our morning coffee.

What can I do to be a better judge of what I read?

Information is power. Brush up your knowledge of human biology and basic nutrition; it will help you become a more discriminating reader. You will soon find that some reports in the popular media sound too good to be true. Look for other reports on the same subject in other publications. Do they all sound the same? That may be because the journalists are too dependent on the same sources of information. They may all attend the same manufacturer's press briefing, for example.

Learn which journalists are best. As a rule, the better the quality of a newspaper or magazine, the higher its standard of technical reporting. If you have doubts, or want more information, ask questions. Write to the manufacturer of a new product. Write to the journalist involved through their publication. Go to the library and ask for help getting facts before you make a major lifestyle change.

Read all new health and medical advice in the media with a certain degree of scepticism. 'Hot' news in the evening paper, or your favourite monthly magazine, about an astounding new medical finding is no reason to immediately alter the way you live. Wait a while, and see what later reports say. Remember that people working in the media need to report news. Stories about health and medical care grab public interest. To hold our attention and excite public interest, journalists may 'hype', or oversimplify, research findings published in the medical literature. By doing so, they may give a misleading impression of the importance and true meaning of its results.

An article by M. Angell, published in the highly regarded scientific journal, *The New England Journal of Medicine,* described how reinterpretation of medical research for the media can alter its importance. It described a situation in which a properly conducted research investigation showed a minor difference in the success rate of two medical treatments following an acute myocardial infarction. When this investigation was reported in the non-scientific press, the wording could have led some readers to believe greater divergence existed between the treatments than was the case. The report in the popular press was technically correct, but the emphasis on the success rate of one drug over the other was misleadingly overstated.

How can I decide what to believe?

Ultimately, believe in your own good judgement. Some medical stories reported in the press sound too good to be true, or just don't make good sense when you stop to think about them. For example, can it be right to try to maintain yourself on a diet totally lacking fat?

Encouraged by articles in the media and attractive advertising campaigns by food manufacturers, an increasing number of people in the United States and elsewhere in westernized countries are striving to eat a totally fat-free diet. Does that make sense? Knowing that fats are a normal part of all life forms, and are found in key nutrients, such as mother's milk, can it be that our health will be improved by totally eliminating them from our diet? Some knowledge of basic biology should lead to a simple answer: No!

On the other hand, years of scientific research pointing to the same conclusion should be heeded. For example, the evidence that smoking cigarettes is harmful to your health – and probably that of everyone around you – is overwhelming.

Good common sense should tell you not to smoke.

Good common sense also tells you to eat a balanced diet, and to avoid going to extremes when adopting new ideas about your health.

SOURCES

M. Angell and J. Kassirer, 'Clinical Research – What Should the Public Believe?', *Nutrition Reviews* (Volume 52, Number 9, pages 320–322, 1994).

H. Applewhite, '*Trans*-isomers, Serum Lipids and Cardiovascular Disease: Another Point of View', *Nutrition Reviews* (Volume 51, Number 11, pages 344–345, 1993).

Julia Child, *The Way to Cook* (Alfred A. Knopf Inc., New York, NY, 1989).

T. P. Coultate, *Food: The Chemistry of its Components*, Second Edition (The Royal Society of Chemistry, Cambridge, 1989 reprinted 1995).

T. P. Coultate and Jill Davies, *Food: The Definitive Guide* (The Royal Society of Chemistry, Cambridge, 1994).

Robert H. Garrison Jr and Elizabeth Somer, *The Nutrition Desk Reference* (Keats Publishing Inc., Connecticut, 1990).

Stanley N. Gershoff, 'Vitamin C (Ascorbic Acid): New Roles, New Requirements?', *Nutrition Reviews* (Volume 51, Number 11, pages 313–326, 1993).

David F. Horrobin, *Omega-6 Essential Fatty Acids: Pathophysiology and Roles in Clinical Medicine* (Wiley-Liss, New York, NY, 1990).

David F. Horrobin, 'Nutritional and Medical Importance of Gamma-linolenic Acids', *Progress in Lipid Research* (Volume 31, Number 2, pages 163–194, 1992).

Larousse *Gastronomique* (Mandarin Octopus, London, 1990).

S. Johnson and F. N. Johnson: Editors, *Gamma Linolenic Acid, Reviews in Contemporary Pharmacotherapy* (Volume 1, Number 1, 1990).

McCance and Widdowson's The Composition of Foods: Fifth Edition (Royal Society of Chemistry and The Ministry of Agriculture, Fisheries and Food, 1991).

'Revising the Dietary Guidelines for Americans', *Nutrition Reviews* (Volume 52, Number 11, pages 394–395, 1994).

E. B. Rimm and others, 'Vitamin E Consumption and the Risk of Coronary Heart Disease in Men', *The New England Journal of Medicine* (Volume 328, Number 20, pages 1450–1456, 1993).

Jenny Salmon, *Dietary Reference Values: A Guide* (Department of Health, HMSO, London, 1991).

M. J. Stamffer and others, 'Vitamin E Consumption and the Risk of Coronary Disease in Women', *The New England Journal of Medicine* (Volume 328, Number 20, pages 1444–1449, 1993).

S. Welch, C. David and A. Shaw. 'A Brief History of Food Guides in the United States', *Nutrition Today* (November/December, pages 6–11, 1992).

Robert Youngson, *The Antioxidant Health Plan: How to Beat the Effects of Free Radicals* (Thorsons/HarperCollins*Publishers*, London, 1994).

INDEX